JHIM

JOURNAL *of*
Healthcare Information Management®

Vol. 13, No. 2, Summer 1999

W9-COJ-772

JOURNAL OF HEALTHCARE INFORMATION MANAGEMENT® (ISSN 1099-811X) is published quarterly by the Healthcare Information and Management Systems Society (HIMSS) and Jossey-Bass Publishers. Subscription to this publication is a benefit of membership in HIMSS. Statements and opinions appearing in articles and departments of the journal are those of the authors and do not necessarily reflect the position of HIMSS.

Note: Starting with Volume 10, Number 1, each volume of Journal of Healthcare Information Management® begins with the Spring issue. Volumes 1–9 began with the Winter issue.

Journal of Healthcare Information Management® is indexed by the American Hospital Association's Hospital Literature Index and HEALTH, a joint database of the AHA and the National Library of Medicine.

TO ORDER subscriptions, single issues, or article reprints, please refer to the Ordering Information page at the back of this issue.

ADDRESS CHANGES: Postmaster: Send to Jossey-Bass Publishers, 350 Sansome Street, San Francisco, CA 94104-1342. HIMSS subscribers: Send to Healthcare Information and Management Systems Society, 230 East Ohio Street, Suite 500, Chicago, IL 60611-3201. Non-HIMSS subscribers: Send to Jossey-Bass Publishers, 350 Sansome Street, San Francisco, CA 94104-1342.

Printed in the United States of America on acid-free recycled paper containing 100 percent recovered waste paper, of which at least 20 percent is post-consumer waste.

CONTENTS

CALL FOR PAPERS
Journal of Healthcare Information Management®
1999–2000 Editorial Calendar

Spring 2000

Topic	Internet
Proposal Deadline	May 1, 1999
Manuscript Deadline	July 1, 1999

Summer 2000

Topic	Emerging Technologies
Proposal Deadline	August 1, 1999
Manuscript Deadline	October 1, 1999

Fall 2000

Topic	Aftermath of Y2K
Proposal Deadline	November 1, 1999
Manuscript Deadline	January 1, 2000

Prospective authors may view the HIMSS Writer's Guidelines at the back of this journal.

EDITOR'S INTRODUCTION

This issue of the *Journal of Healthcare Information Management* focuses on issues surrounding the development and impact of clinical decision support systems (CDSS). This topic is related to many other types of information management systems in healthcare delivery settings. Whether you are in the clinical systems, management engineering, information systems, or telecommunications constituency, you are likely to be involved in some way with a CDSS now or in the near future.

There have been many papers and presentations on different aspects of clinical decision support (CDS) over the years, and a number of useful books are devoted to the subject[1-3] as well as to the impact of healthcare information management in practice.[4] What is increasingly evident, however, is that we now see the widespread adoption of tools for clinical information management in routine practice. As electronic medical record (EMR) systems become widely used, they make available both the data to drive CDSS as well as the vehicle with which to provide CDS to the user. This volume focuses on the essential building blocks for CDSS and reviews the principal application domains of CDS that have had the greatest impact on physician behavior.

The purpose of this volume is to provide the healthcare information management professional with a broad overview of the essential building blocks for CDS and of the principal application domains of CDSS. In the first article Leslie E. Perreault and Jane B. Metzger provide a practical framework for understanding CDS. They review various clinical and financial motivations for CDS and notable implementations of CDSS. Their taxonomy for CDS is useful for delineating the functionality and impact of various systems. They describe useful ways in which CDS may be tailored to the user at the point of care. They also describe how CDSS may be integrated across the continuum of care.

In the second article, Carol A. Broverman addresses the critical standards issues pertaining to the development and implementation of CDSS. The author gives an excellent review of relevant standard setting efforts for knowledge representation and CDS. She reviews progress being made in the HL7 decision support SIG as well as efforts underway within other American National Standards Institute (ANSI) standards-development organizations. There is great promise in the area of standards development for CDS as more robust models emerge for clinical terminology from Systematized Nomenclature of Human Medicine – Reference Terminology (SNOMED-RT) and information modeling from Health Level 7's (HL7) reference information model efforts.

The third, fourth, and fifth articles address key application domains in which providers make innumerable decisions on a daily basis that result in billions of dollars in healthcare expenditures, and may profoundly impact healthcare outcomes: diagnosis, drug ordering, and disease management. Each of these articles focuses on critical issues surrounding the development and impact of CDSS in the chapter's application domain.

In the third article, Eta S. Berner summarizes the principal systems available in the area of diagnostic decision support: DXplain, QMR, Iliad, and Meditel. These systems are designed to support analysis of patient signs and symptoms to produce a differential diagnosis. More often than not, however, they may be most useful as an "electronic textbook" to sort through relationships between patient findings and diseases, and the relationships between diseases themselves. Her article summarizes her own work and that of others, which analyzes the performance of these systems and their impact on clinical care. As the automation of clinical record keeping proceeds in this country, it may be that these systems become more widely adopted when tightly coupled to electronic medical record systems.

The fourth article, by John Poikonen and John M. Leventhal, provide an excellent overview of CDS for medication management at the point of care. The authors review a variety of issues leading to increased costs and clinical information mismanagement related to pharmaceutical issues. They also provide a review of the impact CDSS have had on medication management. Essential features of a medication advising system are then described and the means by which alerts may be delivered to the ordering provider are discussed. They also discuss CDS for formulary management. This chapter gives an excellent overview of codes and structures for pharmaceuticals and how they may be used in CDSS.

The fifth article describes disease management and the developments that have led to this area of CDS. Rufus S. Howe, Michael B. Terpening, and Sandeep Wadhwa offer an integrated view of total quality management and its relationship to CDS. They define disease management in practical terms and identify various stakeholders and technology components to enable a successful disease management program. In their view of the future, the authors see an environment supporting secure data sharing with maintenance of patient confidentiality to improve physician-driven disease management and ultimately patient-centered disease management.

Subsequent articles focus on the implementation of CDSS in different healthcare settings or environments. The sixth article focuses on CDS in ambulatory settings. J. Marc Overhage, William M. Tierney, and Clement J. McDonald provide an excellent overview of critical functionality in CDS for outpatient environments. They review essential design criteria to make CDSS work in the highly dynamic outpatient environment. Various insights are given from the rich experience at the Regenstrief Institute for Healthcare regarding how to tailor CDS for clinicians at the point of care. They describe the Regenstrief Medical Record System (RMRS) and the impact it has had on a variety of care practices in the outpatient environment at Indiana University. The authors describe future trends in outpatient order management including improved user modeling to guide the content, form, and structure of an advisory at the point of care.

The seventh and eighth articles focus on CDS in the inpatient environment. In the seventh article Gilad J. Kuperman, Dean F. Sittig, and M. Michael Shabot describe some of the best known and effective examples of CDSS. Many of the early trials of CDS technology occurred in hospital environments. In their historical review, the authors describe how these systems arose and how some are in routine use today in modern hospitals. The authors also provide a practical and accurate review of the many issues relating to the successful design and implementation of a complicated knowledge-based CDSS, including applicable standards, technology, support and maintenance issues, and knowledge engineering. They also provide a useful taxonomy to distinguish among the various types of knowledge-based CDSS: *formatting applications* that present the data in a more useful way, *interpreting applications* for a single clinical data element or observation, full *consultation applications* for diagnostic or therapeutic CDS, *monitoring applications* that can alert providers to critical events, and *critiquing applications* that may provide critical feedback to a user's patient management plan.

In the eighth article Jonathan M. Teich gives an excellent review of approaches to Physician Order Entry (POE). Dr. Teich describes the importance of POE as a focal point for CDS. The vast majority of healthcare costs arise from physician's orders for their patients. Teich describes the ways in which physicians can be supported at the time of order entry and reviews the impact CDS for order entry has had in a variety of academic environments. Teich reviews essential attributes of successful CDSS for order entry as well as governance and review structures that must be in place to manage the knowledge engineering and implementation process for these CDSS. Teich also reviews functional aspects of CDS for order entry including order sets, recurring orders and various specific functional components including structured ordering, substitute therapy checking, parameter checking, excessive utilization checking, time-based checking, and other techniques. The impact of CDS at the time of POE can be dramatic and Teich gives several highlights.

In the ninth article, Homer R. Warner, Jr., Di Guo, Christopher Mason, William Harty, and Lili Li describe a novel architectural approach that is provided to demonstrate integration of all the prior concepts presented in this volume in an effort to provide CDS across the continuum of care. The authors describe an interesting application design for CDS and describe the clinical event monitor that is built as an autonomous decision support application feeding off of HL7 messages in a clinical information management environment. The CEM "listens" to HL7 messages and interprets them on the basis of a large rule-oriented knowledge base of clinical information. Should rules fire prompting an alert, alerts may be delivered to providers via a variety of modalities (e-mail or page for example). An interesting feature of this design is that it leaves legacy systems in the environment untouched but nevertheless provides a variety of essential decision support features. Alerts may be tailored to individual users not only by method of delivery but also by severity, current covering physician relationships, as well as coding of "do not repeat" alert until certain criteria are satisfied. The authors describe the implementation of the clinical event monitor in two environments and describe its hardware requirements as well.

These are indeed exciting times we live in. Healthcare is the largest sector of the United States economy, and we are in the midst of profound change in the organization of the healthcare delivery system, and the technology used to support it. CDS is one of the more exciting areas of change being driven by the need for ever-more-efficient and effective healthcare services. For all members of HIMSS, in any constituency, it is likely CDS systems, in one form or another, will become a bigger part of our lives.

BLACKFORD MIDDLETON, MD, MPH, MSc
SENIOR VICE PRESIDENT FOR CLINICAL INFORMATICS
MEDICALOGIC, INC.

References

1. Berner, E. S. "Clinical Decision Support Systems: Theory and Practice." In K. J. Hannah and M. J. Ball (eds.), *Health Informatics.* New York: Springer, 1999.
2. Dick, R. S., Steen, E. B., and Detmer, D. E. "The Computer-Based Patient Record: An Essential Technology for Healthcare." Washington, D.C.: National Academy Press, 1997.
3. Todd, W. E., and Nash, D. *Disease Management: A Systems Approach to Improving Patient Outcomes.* Chicago: American Hospital Publishing, Inc., 1997.
4. Millenson, M. L. *Demanding Medical Excellence: Doctors and Accountability in the Information Age.* Chicago: University of Chicago Press, 1997.

A Pragmatic Framework for Understanding Clinical Decision Support

Leslie E. Perreault, Jane B. Metzger

The Institute of Medicine, in its 1991 report on the computer-based patient record (CPR), emphasized clinical decision support (CDS) as an essential component of a CPR and a major reason for managing patient information electronically.[1] As health care faces continued pressure to deliver appropriate care and effectively manage the care process in and across increasingly complex settings, the belief is growing that CDS is a desirable and even necessary capability. Supporting this belief is an increasing body of experience and research showing that clinical decision support systems (CDSS), appropriately implemented, can improve the quality of care, reduce costs, and improve patient satisfaction. More and more institutions—academic health centers, community-based organizations, and physician group practices alike—are actively pursuing the goal of implementing patient-care systems that include CDS, backing their plans with significant investments of capital and staff resources.

Among the many motivations for implementing CDSS are these:

Improving patient care—alerting staff to critical values, potential drug interactions, and allergies

Reducing costs—controlling medication orders and avoiding duplicate or unnecessary tests

Disseminating expert knowledge—supporting clinical diagnosis and treatment-plan processes, facilitating adoption of guidelines for disease and wellness management, communicating best practices, and enabling population-based management

Managing clinical complexity—keeping patients on research and chemotherapy protocols

Monitoring clinical details—tracking orders and referrals with no results, need for follow-up, and need for preventive services

Managing administrative complexity—supporting clinical coding and documentation, procedures authorization, and referrals management

Educating students and residents—suggesting areas of investigation, critiquing plans, and displaying explanations and relevant references

Supporting clinical research—identifying patients who may fit a clinical protocol and assisting in management of those patients in accordance with protocols

Definitions of CDS by individuals, health organizations, and vendors vary widely. We as an industry have decided that we want CDS, yet there is little agreement on what it is. This confusion is understandable given the complexity and multidimensional nature of CDS and the varied ancestry of today's systems. Many of the earliest CDS applications were developed as stand-alone expert systems to support specific aspects of medical decision making such as differential diagnosis or therapy planning (for example, Quick Medical Reference and DXPlain). Institutionwide CDSS for generating clinical reminders and alerts were initially developed at a small number of institutions such as LDS Hospital in Salt Lake City, the Regenstrief Institute for Healthcare in Indianapolis, Brigham and Women's Hospital in Boston, and Columbia-Presbyterian Medical Center in New York City. These and other clinical informatics initiatives continue today, and they have created a foundation for commercial systems development. An increasing number of commercial software vendors now offer patient-care systems that include CDS. Many of the most familiar CDSS assist clinicians in caring for individual patients. CDS systems also have a legacy, however, in traditional (financially oriented) decision-support systems. As clinical data beyond diagnosis and procedure codes are captured and stored in data warehouses, traditional decision-support systems have been extended to enable retrospective analysis of population-based data, thereby helping care providers understand and improve clinical practice.

In its broadest sense, a CDSS can be any automated tool that helps clinicians improve the delivery or management of patient care. In its ideal sense, CDS is a set of knowledge-based tools that are fully integrated with both the clinician workflow components of a CPR and a repository of complete and accurate clinical data. Neither view is particularly useful for an organization that is trying to develop a CDS capability from scratch or to compare alternative approaches or commercial products.

An organization considering new investments in CDS must answer practical questions such as these:

What types of decision support will provide the most value?

How much should we invest, and what value will we gain?

Do we have the necessary technical infrastructure (data repository, standard clinical vocabulary, network, workstations) and organizational infrastructure (clinician leadership, executive commitment, funding) to support CDS implementation and ongoing deployment?

Without a clear definition of the task to be accomplished, answers to these questions will remain elusive, and the magnitude of the endeavor may be overwhelming.

The purpose of this article is to present a pragmatic framework for understanding and deploying CDSS. Using this framework, we expose a multidimensional spectrum of CDS capabilities and deconstruct CDS into component functions. Such a deconstruction helps to counter a common view of CDS as an all-or-nothing capstone to clinical-systems implementation. The framework is a useful tool for matching organizational objectives with specific CDS projects that can provide value, either individually or in concert. It may also assist in matching CDS functions with specific organizational and technical prerequisites, thus helping organizations target appropriate goals and gain more immediate value from their CDS investments than they otherwise might.

Our CDS framework covers systems that support care providers in their direct interactions with and decision making about patients. Although broad in scope, this perspective is not all-encompassing. For example, we have not included automated systems that assist in waveform interpretation or analysis of radiology or pathology images. For now, our definition also excludes decision-support tools designed for use by patients, administrators, employers, and other noncare providers.

Dimensions of Clinical Decision Support

The rich and varied nature of CDSS designed for use by clinicians engaged in direct patient care is apparent in Table 1, which identifies eighteen dimensions of CDS. In creating a CDS vision and specific project plans, an organization must carefully consider who will be the focus of decision making and when, what types of CDS capabilities to implement first, where to deploy the tools, and how, from a technical perspective, they will be implemented.

Who is the focus of the decision? These parameters address basic questions of approach and scope. The decision focus indicates whether the CDSS is designed to assist in caring for a particular patient or in understanding and improving clinical practices. The target population addresses implementation scope. Is the system relevant to all patients or to a population subset such as health-plan members, full-risk (capitated) patients, or specific high-risk patients (for example, those with diabetes or congestive heart failure)?

Where will the system be used? The earliest institutionwide CDSS were deployed in the inpatient setting. These systems were typically associated with medication orders processed in pharmacy systems, the components of physician order entry in a hospital information system, and reports of laboratory-test results. Early CDS efforts in ambulatory care were focused on prescription processing (drug-drug and drug-allergy checking) and simple reminders concerning health-maintenance interventions. As healthcare organizations move to provide population-based care (disease, demand, and other

Table 1. Dimensions of Clinical Decision Support

Who?/When?	What?	Where?	How?
Decision focus (patient care, practice improvement) Target population (single patient, member population, capitated patients, high-risk patients) Timing (concurrent or retrospective)	Decision context (medical decision, care-management decision) Decision type (assessment, diagnosis, planning, alerting) Degree of customization to a clinical context (generic tailored, customized) Complexity/sophistication of logic (single dimension, multiple dimensions) Mode of interaction (recommending/advising, coaching, critiquing) Level of interplay (static, dynamic/interactive) Trigger types (user-invoked, data-driven, event-driven, time/expectation driven) Knowledge-representation/ inference method (rules, medical-logic modules/ Arden Syntax, neural network, decision tree, clinical algorithm) Extent of integration with external knowledge sources (embedded-expert system, information-retrieval systems)	Scope of use (single setting, multiple setting, cross-continuum) Care-coordination focus (encounter, episode, disease course) System users (local users, designated users, enterprise access) System access (local, enterprise, remote, or Internet access)	Data integration (stand-alone, linked to data repository) Workflow integration (stand-alone, embedded in application)

cross-continuum care management), we are defining new requirements for information capture and management, as well as new opportunities for CDS.[2] The scope of use indicates whether the CDSS is designed for use in a single setting (inpatient unit, ambulatory-care clinic, intensive-care unit) or whether its functions span settings across the continuum of care. The care-coordination focus identifies whether the decision support is encounter-based or spans an episode or disease course. User access identifies the CDS system's user base (limited to specific providers associated with a facility or program or accessible to all providers). System access specifies where and how the system can be accessed (for example, local versus remote access). Organizations considering deployment of CDSS should clearly understand their clinical-management goals, then determine an appropriate CDS type and implementation venue.

What are the design features of the system? From a user perspective, the critical dimensions of a CDS relate to what the system does and how it functions. The decision context for many CDS projects has shifted over time from support for specific medical decisions (for example, what is the most likely diagnosis?) to support for care management (for example, what plan for care will result in the best clinical outcome while avoiding unnecessary costs?). The degree of customization to the clinical context (discussed below) is an important factor in clinician acceptance and system value, and it also has substantial implications for cost, difficulty of implementation, and required level of user-system interaction. Other dimensions of CDS function include the complexity of the medical logic, the knowledge representation (rules, neural networks, decision trees), the level of interplay between system and user (static or interactive), and the types of triggering events (user-invoked, data-driven, time-driven). Healthcare organizations should evaluate the sophistication of a potential CDSS's function relative to the availability of clinical resources (interest, expertise) for system implementation, testing, and ongoing maintenance.

How does the system fit into the technical architecture? A robust technical infrastructure is a prerequisite for the most sophisticated forms of CDS: highly interactive, customized CDSS that are integrated with clinical applications and workflow. To implement such systems, an organization must first have implemented a repository for complete and accurate clinical data, a consistent clinical-data model and clinical vocabulary, and high-quality patient-care information systems. These capabilities determine the extent to which a CDSS is integrated with clinical data (requiring users to reenter data or allowing them to access data in a clinical-data repository) and the extent of integration with the workflow (stand-alone application or integration with the clinical support tasks of documenting, ordering, planning, and reviewing results and outcomes). The stand-alone nature of many early CDSS was recognized as a barrier to their acceptance. Today, building up the technical foundation (particularly the necessary data capture and management) remains a rate-limiting step in implementing CDSS that are fully integrated with online patient records.

Continuum of Clinical Decision Support

Given the spectrum of choices described in the preceding section, it is no wonder that many organizations experience confusion in defining specific CDS objectives and determining an implementation approach. These choices, however, will have major implications for cost, difficulty of implementation, physician acceptance, and the magnitude of benefits that can be achieved. To help in understanding the range of CDSS, we have developed a high-level framework that represents a continuum of CDS approaches (Figure 1). We classify CDSS in four general categories: access to information, guided choices, knowledge-based prompting, and understanding clinical practice.

Access to Information. The most basic form of decision support is providing easy access to general or patient-specific clinical data and information. CDS capabilities in this category are aimed at delivering the right information at the right time and place to enable informed clinical decision making. We have ample evidence that information deficiencies contribute to errors of omission and commission. Furthermore, we now have sufficient experience with advanced patient-care systems to know that a system's usefulness to clinicians can be enhanced by integrating and presenting information in different ways depending on the clinical context. For these reasons, efforts to improve information access and maximize the value of information are important foundation tactics for improving clinical decisions.

Guided Choice. Guided choices provide a second level of support for clinical decision making. CDS capabilities in this category are designed to make it easy for care providers to make the "right" choices among available options. Implicit in the concept of guided choice are the ideas of preferred alternatives and standards of care. These tools may reflect professional, departmental, or organizational norms or guidelines. Typical forms of guided choice include templates, default values, and menus of options for ordering interventions or structuring documentation. More sophisticated systems may tie the alternatives

Figure 1. A Continuum of Clinical Decision Support

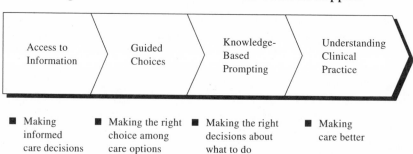

that are presented to an underlying clinical guideline or pathway. An organization may adopt either a passive or active stance with respect to guided choices. Guided-choice functions may subtly reinforce desired practices by making them relatively easy to select (for example, presenting preferred antibiotics in a favorites list). Enforcement of desired behaviors (for example, by eliminating certain options) is a more active use of guided choice.

Knowledge-Based Prompting. Knowledge-based prompting, the third level of CDS, is designed to actively assist clinicians in making the right care decisions. These CDS tools help to determine the correct clinical diagnosis in planning therapy or by alerting the clinician to relevant important information (for example, laboratory panic value or potential drug interaction). Whereas the knowledge and policies behind guided choices are typically embedded in a system's design and presentation, knowledge-based prompting systems usually have explicit rules (or other knowledge representation) and inference mechanisms. These systems require a strong infrastructure of both technology (repository, medical-entities dictionary) and organization (physician leadership and active participation).

Understanding Clinical Practice. Understanding clinical practice, the fourth level of CDS, transcends the here and now of a particular clinical interaction. CDS capabilities in this category are aimed at achieving overall improvement in care delivery. These CDSS are population-focused and used retrospectively to identify patterns and trends, which in turn can be used to guide future decisions, identify current best practices, and evaluate and refine clinical guidelines. This function is inextricably tied to clinician-directed CDS because it provides the insight necessary for identifying opportunities to reduce variation or avoid errors. These insights are also needed to support ongoing refinement of CDS. In addition, retrospective analysis is a prerequisite for giving clinical-practice feedback to providers to reinforce desired practice behaviors.

Forms and Delivery Mechanisms for Clinical Decision Support

Using the definitions and the high-level framework described above, we created a matrix framework for classifying the many CDS forms and delivery mechanisms. This framework, shown in Table 2, organizes the many dimensions of CDS; it can be used to classify the different capabilities and to analyze their diffusion into clinical practice. The four columns correspond to the levels of CDS shown in Figure 1. The rows depict the specificity of support to the clinical context, a major differentiating feature. Looking at the state of the art, we identified three categories of match:

Generic—requiring user selection or focus to obtain support relevant to the care situation at hand

Table 2. A Framework for Understanding the Forms and Delivery Mechanisms of Clinical Decision Support

Level of Match with Clinical Context	Access to Information	Guided Choices	Knowledge-Based Prompting	Understanding Clinical Practice
Generic	Institutional-knowledge access by query (guidelines, policies) Domain-knowledge access by query (research literature) Patient-data access by query (single results)	Common calculations (user query) Common choices (by discipline, by user) Template-based documentation (user selection from predetermined choices)	Notification by user request (passive) User notification if in patient record or application Trigger by event Uniform priority of alerts/reminders	Basic categorization of patients, providers for aggregate analysis (provider, specialty, patient age/sex, disease-related group) Outlier identification/ provider profiling Compliance with clinical pathway/ guideline Delivery-process analysis (cycle times, success rates, retention rates)
Tailored	Indexed and searchable knowledge access (relevant topics) Trend analysis of patient data (single results over time) Integrated patient-data views (latest results, by encounter, tailored to provider) Stat print/auto-fax of abnormal results	Order-linked calculator (autodisplay) Order sets Display of common defaults in orders Template-based documentation (guided by decision rules with branching logic) Order-elements display with preferred choices (clinical rules, payer rules)	Team support (routing to team) Alert escalation (user or location) User notification if signed onto system Trigger by specific patient-data value User-set, timed reminder Variable notification routing (based on mode for recipient)	Severity-adjusted analysis of aggregate performance in care Variance analysis— simple pathways/ guidelines Drill-down capability (based on classification criteria)

Customized	Highlighted display of abnormal results (user query)	Shortcut to knowledge access (case-relevant)	Display of linked appropriateness criteria (order or referral)	Variable notification routing (system-specified)	Severity-adjusted analysis of aggregate performance in care based on clinical characteristics such as comorbidity

Customized

Highlighted display of abnormal results (user query)
Results tracking by review status (viewed, signed)
Shortcut to knowledge access (case-relevant)
Trend analysis of patient data (multiple parameters)
Integrated patient-data views (by chronic disease, by problem, by clinical context)
Results bundling by encounter (batch for review when all completed)
Results linked to patient-specific correspondence

Display of linked appropriateness criteria (order or referral)
Order sets linked with clinical paths/time-based care plans
Individualized visit planning (interventions due for user selection)
Outreach work lists of patients with interventions due
Time-based care plan linked to population risk group

Variable notification routing (system-specified)
Priority-ranked display of alerts/reminders
Coverage list (notification, routing)
Alert escalation (no response, user-specified)
Alert of nonuser (pager or other mode for notification)
Time-driven trigger
Alert linked to corrective action
Alert correction because of new information
User-selected customization of delivery options
Display of alerts/reminders based on relevance to clinical context
Stand-alone expert system for interactive use

Severity-adjusted analysis of aggregate performance in care based on clinical characteristics such as comorbidity
Variance analysis—complex (combined) pathways/guidelines
Drill-down capability (patient level)

Tailored—focused on the clinical context in terms of basic dimensions such as
   type of decision or type of provider
Customized—focused on the clinical context in accordance with multiple
   dimensions reflecting the patient-specific situation and the type of decision

We next assembled information on forms and delivery mechanisms from various sources including the clinical informatics literature; research publications emanating from development sites with self-developed, advanced patient-care systems; recent conversations with major vendors offering CDS as part of commercially available software; and requests for proposals for advanced clinical systems prepared by First Consulting Group associates in recent consulting engagements. To that collection of available and desirable capabilities we added a small number of items identified in our recent research on deploying practice guidelines for disease and wellness management.

   Access to Information. The access to information category includes all forms and mechanisms whereby information is made available to the clinician. We have included domain and institutional information in addition to patient-specific information because these resources—structured as guidelines or protocols or access to research evidence—can assist clinicians in reaching decisions about their patients.

   At the generic level, information resources are passive, and the clinician must initiate a system query to access desired information. In the next level, information obtained by query can be integrated and displayed in formats such as graphs or flow sheets, which provide a view of trends over time, and patient-at-a-glance displays, which integrate many types of information. We have also included some forms of assistance to the clinician in managing information according to urgency or to normal or abnormal diagnostic findings.

   Customized capabilities include facilitated access to knowledge, such as research literature, as a clinician is ordering a medication with complex dosing or suggested secondary orders. We consider this customized because the knowledge made accessible is pertinent to the particular clinical decision being made for a particular patient. This group also includes more complex, integrated data views—trends in multiple parameters and patient-data views organized by chronic disease, problem, or clinical context (emergency unit, intensive-care unit). Two capabilities aid clinicians in managing their review of results (bundling all for an encounter so they can be reviewed at once) and response (patient correspondence).

   Guided Choices. At the generic level, decision-support tools are passive (users must seek them out). The ability to access tools for common calculations and to select interventions (such as medications) from a list of common choices clearly makes it easier (and often faster) to initiate the desired intervention correctly. We have also included simple documentation templates in which users select from predetermined choices.

Support for the ordering function steps up a level with order sets (guiding the clinician to multiple recommended orders for a clinical context, such as admission or a particular condition or both, and to preoperative orders for a particular surgical procedure). The calculator (for dosing, for example) is automatically displayed when clinicians are writing relevant orders and is set up for the particular inputs (for example, patient weight) and calculation needed for the medication in question. We have also included orders for which the recommended choices are displayed first or highlighted to alert the clinician to clinical appropriateness rules developed by the institution or payer-driven rules such as medication formulary. Another variation on this approach is the display of a reminder message concerning appropriateness considerations as the clinician enters the order. At this level, template-based documentation is guided by decision rules and branching logic based on patient-specific information available at each branch. This type of guidance more closely mimics the thought process of the clinician than simple templates (and can also speed the entry of documentation).

Further customization of order sets involves linkage with a clinical pathway or (more typical for disease management in ambulatory care) a time-based care plan. When a clinician activates the pathway, order sets for the current time period of the pathway are launched.

We have encountered two varieties of guided choices fairly recently as part of self-developed information-technology support for population-based disease and wellness management.[3 4 5] Visit plans, which can be either a computer-generated printout or a display, detail interventions that are being tracked for the patient and are due (blood-pressure check, HbA1c testing). These reminders aid the clinician in making the most of each visit, including times when the patient is seen for another or an acute problem. A related tool is an outreach work list, which helps clinicians identify patients being tracked for disease management who have not been seen and have interventions due.

Knowledge-Based Prompting. Many of the capabilities for knowledge-based prompting relate to triggers for prompts and methods of notification. At the generic level, triggers are events such as a scheduled visit, and notification is relatively passive. Users either select the option to review reminders or are alerted to messages about a patient if they are reviewing that patient's electronic record. A variation of the review mode alerts clinician users when they are signed on to the application (such as an electronic medical record). At this level, alerts and reminders are handled uniformly regardless of urgency or the content of the message.

More tailored prompting is triggered by new patient data (for example, a laboratory result) or user-set, timed reminders (either a personal tickler file or a message routed to another user). Notification capabilities can include escalation (to a user or location) and variable routing based on user (for example, fax to one physician, electronic message to another who is a system user) or system-specified by parameters such as urgency and patient location.

Notification of clinical team members is another feature that may be available, especially in acute care. Alerts and reminders can be priority-ranked and routed differently depending on the importance of a timely response. At this level, users are notified if they are signed on to the system (not necessarily the patient-care application).

Customized approaches include the ability to notify clinicians when they are not using the computer system via pager, for example. Advanced designs incorporate a coverage list (clinician covering the service), escalation when alert messages are not successfully delivered within a requisite time period, and user-selected customization of delivery modes for notifications. Triggers can be time-driven and can notify the clinician of nonoccurrence of planned interventions (for example, the patient is a no-show for a scheduled visit with a therapist or fails to pick up a refill for a prescribed medication). Other advanced features include the ability to amend prior alerts and reminders when new patient information (such as an amended laboratory result) requires different advice and the ability to selectively display (turn off) prompts based on relevance to the clinical context (for example, no reminders concerning overdue health-maintenance interventions for patients in the hospital).

Also included at the customized level are stand-alone expert systems that aid the clinician in reaching a decision about diagnosis or treatment. Generally these are independent of a patient-care application and patient database, and the clinician interactively enters patient-specific information needed by the program. These systems deliver advice in a different way in that the clinician must be actively seeking advice and the CDS tool is not integrated with a clinical application. However, we included these systems in the customized level because the resulting advice is highly customized to the patient.

Understanding Clinical Practice. Retrospective decision support is another important component of a concerted effort to reduce undesirable variation in treatment and outcomes because it serves two critical purposes: it provides insight into care processes and practices so that improvement opportunities can be identified, including targets for CDS; and it can be provided to individual clinicians to reinforce desired behavior in the clinical management of their patients.

Generic capabilities include the traditional approaches of outlier identification and provider profiling and basic patient groupings for analysis of practice patterns (typically using discharge or billing information or both). Another capability at this basic level is the ability to analyze compliance with clinical pathways or guidelines and, when the information is available, to gain insight into care processes. Examples of such information include cycle times, length of stay, complication rates, and retention rates.

Another form of retrospective analysis is the ability to adjust patient groupings to account for differences in the clinical status of patients. At the tailored level this is accomplished using severity adjustment within individual disease states. This differentiation becomes much more refined when more clinical parameters (such as comorbidity) can be accommodated in the severity adjustment. Variance analysis—usually applied to analysis involving clinical pathways and time-based care plans—is simple at the tailored level but incorporates more combinations of patient-specific circumstances at the customized level.

The power of retrospective clinical decision support has another dimension, which we have not incorporated into this framework: the data set available for analysis. This set determines what types of hypotheses can be examined—in terms of both the number of patient-specific elements available to the CDS and the types and settings of care situations. To date much of the retrospective analysis has been confined to acute care, with outcomes such as length of stay predominating, because of data limitations.

Diffusion of Clinical Decision Support into Practice

CDS has not been widely implemented in practice. A 1996 study commissioned by the Canadian government surveyed developers of CDS tools and found that only 24 percent of CDSS were actually being used. The top barriers cited in this study were the need for further development; problems with the database, knowledge base, or rule base; output quality; incomplete evaluation; and user interface.[6]

Based on contacts with vendors of commercial patient-care systems, a literature review, and our firm's work in systems implementation, we have estimated the diffusion of CDS using the following categories:

Widely implemented: generally available in commercial patient-care applications that have been implemented in a large number of institutions
Commercially available/some implementation: capabilities available in one or more commercial products to support patient care (at least in alpha or beta implementation)
Experimental: available only in an institution with a self-developed patient-care system or a design feature in development by a commercial vendor
Future: no identified systems but on the wish list for the future

Using these categories, we re-sorted all the entries from Table 2 to create Table 3. In sheer numbers of capabilities, we have made the most progress with access to information and understanding clinical practice. It is encouraging, however, that so many capabilities are available in the early implementations of commercial systems; we can expect further deployment as more organizations implement advanced patient-care systems.

In Table 3 we have also noted (with footnotes) capabilities for which current implementation is largely for one type of clinical situation. For many, predominant implementation is in the acute-care setting or involves mostly laboratory test results (or both). Another rapidly growing concentration of

Table 3. Diffusion of Clinical Decision Support in Practice

Implementation Status	Access to Information	Guided Choices	Knowledge-Based Prompting	Understanding Clinical Practice
Widely implemented	Institutional-knowledge access by query (guidelines, policies) Domain-knowledge access by query (research literature) Patient-data access by query (single results)* Indexed and searchable knowledge access (relevant topics) Trend analysis of patient data (single results over time)*† Stat print/auto-fax of abnormal results*†	Common calculations (user query) Common choices (by discipline, by user)# Template-based documentation (user selection from predetermined choices)# Order sets*~	Notification by user request (passive) User notification if in patient record or application# Trigger by event# Uniform priority of alerts/reminders	Basic categorization of patients, providers for aggregate analysis (provider, specialty, patient age/sex, disease-related group)* Outlier identification/provider profiling* Drill-down capability (based on classification criteria)
Commercially available/some implementation	Integrated patient-data views (latest results, by encounter, tailored to provider) Results tracking by review status (results in in-box viewed, signed)† Trend analysis of patient data (multiple parameters) Results bundling by encounter (batch for review when all completed) Results linked to patient-specific correspondence	Order-linked calculator (autodisplay)* Template-based documentation (given by decision rules with branching logic)# Order-elements display with preferred choices (clinical rules, payer rules)# Order sets linked with clinical paths/time-based care plans* Display of linked appropriateness criteria (order or referral)	Alert escalation (user or location) User notification if signed onto system Trigger by specific patient-data value User-set, time reminder# Variable notification routing (based on mode for recipient)# Stand-alone expert system for interactive use	Compliance with clinical pathway/guideline* Severity-adjusted analysis of aggregate performance in care* Delivery-process analysis (cycle times, success rates, retention rates)* Variance analysis—simple pathways/guidelines*

Experimental	Integrated patient-data views (by chronic disease, by problem, by clinical context)	Display of common defaults in orders Time based care plan linked to population risk group Individualized visit planning (interventions due for user selection) Outreach work lists of patients with interventions due	Team support (routing to team)* Variable notification routing (system-specified) Priority-ranked display of alerts/reminders# Coverage list (notification routing)* Alert of nonuser (pager or other mode for notification)* Alert linked to corrective action* Alert correction because of new information* Display of alerts/reminders based on relevance to clinical context Time-driven trigger Alert escalation (no response, user-specified) User-selected customization of delivery options	Variance analysis—(combined) pathways/guidelines* Drill-down capability (patient level)
Future	Shortcut to knowledge access (case-relevant)			Severity-adjusted analysis of aggregate performance in care based on clinical characteristics such as comorbidity

* = primarily in acute care setting. † = primarily in ambulatory care setting. ~ = order transcription more common than physician order entry. # = primarily laboratory results. # = primarily in ambulatory care setting.

deployed tools is in ambulatory-care, rule-based prompting, typically including checking drug and allergy interactions associated with prescription entry and tracking health-maintenance interventions (for example, mammography).

Conclusions

Clearly we have only just begun to apply CDS and to recognize the value of these systems. Through the experiences of pioneering institutions we are beginning to assemble concrete evidence of the benefits of CDSS for improved patient care and reduced costs. We also have recognized a number of challenges to CDS deployment, including the need for extensive and costly foundation clinical systems, development and adoption of consistent data models and clinical vocabulary, active engagement of clinical leadership, and changes to the culture of medical practice. Capturing all desired patient data in coded, electronic form (available to CDS) is particularly difficult when we are dealing with ambulatory-practice data in general and is especially problematic with respect to recording history and physical and progress notes. As an industry, we have reached the point where many organizations buy into the goal of automated support for clinical decision making, but the monetary and staff investments may seem prohibitive in light of the soft evidence on benefits and the long period of investment before returns begin.

For many information-systems and clinical practitioners, the value of CDS may seem obvious, and ongoing debates regarding value are frustrating. Nonetheless, given the enormous sustained investment and organizational commitment required to implement these systems, and the backdrop of tight budgets, cost cutting, and competing initiatives, it is fair to ask, What do we get for what we invest? Describing CDS only as fully integrated, knowledge-based systems can render CDS projects too large or ill-defined for comfortable assessment and, in the process, may delay or preclude investments that can provide immediate value. We believe that by viewing CDS as a toolbox of component capabilities rather than as the "ultimate" clinical application, organizations will be better prepared to match specific objectives with anticipated benefits and appropriate investments. By teasing apart CDS into component capabilities, a health care institution can launch a portfolio of CDS activities— investing in less sophisticated capabilities that are easier to implement and that provide more immediate benefits, as well as in more sophisticated capabilities that require larger investments and ultimately may yield greater value.

Collectively, we have created an ambitious agenda for CDS through medical informatics research goals, vendor product plans, and provider wants. By viewing CDS as a set of component capabilities rather than as a holistic application, we will be better prepared to understand whether we need (and can afford) all of the possible CDS capability and under what circumstances.

References

1. Dick, R. S., and Steen, E. B. (eds.). *The Computer-Based Patient Record: An Essential Technology for Health Care.* Washington, D.C.: National Academy Press, 1997.
2. Metzger, J. B. "Cross-Continuum Care Management: Information Management Challenges." *Strategies for Integrated Health Care.* San Francisco: Jossey-Bass, 1999.
3. Heiser, N. A., and St. Peter, R. F. "Improving the Delivery of Clinical Preventive Services to Women in Managed Care Organizations: A Case Study Analysis." *JCAHO Journal on Quality Improvement,* 1997, *23* (10), 529–549.
4. Friedman, N. M., Gleeson, J. M., Kent, M. J., Foris, M., and Rodriguez, D. J. "Management of Diabetes Mellitus in the Lovelace Health Systems' Episodes of Care Program." *Effective Clinical Practice,* 1998, *1* (1), 5–11.
5. McCulloch, D. K., Price, M. J., Hindmarsh, M., and Wagner, E. H. "A Population-Based Approach to Diabetes Management in a Primary Care Setting: Early Results and Lessons Learned." *Effective Clinical Practice,* 1998, *1* (1), 12–22.
6. Fisher, P., Hollander, M. J., MacKenzie, T., Kleinstiver, P., Sladecek, I., and Peterson, G. "Decision Support Tools in Health Care." In *Making Decisions. Evidence and Information.* Quebec: Editions MultiMondes, 1998.

About the Authors

Leslie E. Perreault is a director with First Consulting Group's Emerging Practices Institute in New York City.

Jane B. Metzger is a vice president with First Consulting Group's Emerging Practices Institute in Boston.

Standards for Clinical Decision Support Systems

Carol A. Broverman, Ph.D.

Clinical decision support systems (CDSS) have long been regarded as a desirable feature of healthcare information systems. In fact, CDSS are often regarded as the carrot that will serve as the reward for clinicians as they weather the cultural changes required to adopt and populate the electronic medical record. CDSS involve the manipulation and leveraging of painstakingly collected clinical data into useful knowledge to assist clinicians in their fundamental practice. CDSS are often advocated to filter, interpret, and flag relevant data to support clinical decision making. Decision-support systems often use rules derived from algorithms, artificial intelligence, or fuzzy logic to assist healthcare professionals in determining the "proper" course of action. The application of CDSS techniques has value both retrospectively across populations and episodes of care and at the point of care in a more patient-focused setting. Much work in CDSS has focused on providing alerts and reminders, while newer systems are targeted at the implementation of more complex protocols of plans of care.

Another type of decision-support system that is important to healthcare enterprises today is executive decision-support systems (EDSS), which extracts data from other systems so that care processes can be analyzed and reworked in order to reduce costs and improve quality of care. Data warehouses and their associated decision-support systems enable healthcare organizations to "mine" data to prospectively re-engineer the clinical process, establish comparable data to evaluate practice patterns, and use outcomes to create cost and quality-conscious best practices. A number of products available today deal with this type of application. While standards for clinical terminology are particularly important for EDSS "data mining," this paper focuses on standardization work that is being applied to patient-centered, integrated CDSS.

Generally speaking, CDSS provide the right information at the right time to the right person in order to facilitate sound and timely clinical judgements. This is a broad definition by design. Many architectural and design variations are employed to provide decision-support behavior within clinical systems, depending on the desired function and the host-system requirements.

Types of Clinical Decision Support Systems

The following distinctions can be made regarding types of CDSS:

Passive versus *active* systems: Passive systems are invoked by users, while active systems perform functions continuously as a by-product of data management. Active decision-support systems that operate seamlessly in the background are more likely to gain acceptance, yet users want to feel that they are in control of the system's behavior.

Aggregate versus *individual, patient-based* systems. Some CDSS analyze patterns across a patient population; other systems analyze data for one patient at a time. Both types of systems are useful depending on the application. Aggregate analyses often form the basis for cost-benefit studies; these results, in turn, can be used as input for devising rules that are leveraged during the treatment of an individual patient who has a profile that has been identified as being of clinical interest.

Concurrent versus *retrospective* systems. Some systems provide feedback concurrent with care giving, while others provide feedback after events have occurred. Wherever possible, concurrency is desirable, as suggestions are interleaved with actual clinical workflow, and the necessity of undoing inadvisable actions after the fact can be avoided.

Systems *integrated with the patient database* versus *stand-alone* systems. Some systems are integrated with a full electronic patient record; stand-alone systems make decisions in a more isolated context or rely on user-supplied information. Integrated systems are more difficult to implement but will be more easily accepted as they are synergistic with workflow and avoid redundant data entry.

Proprietary versus *standards-based* encoding. Some systems use proprietary coding schemes for patient data, rules, and clinical concepts, while other systems adopt industry standards where available and appropriate. A standards-based solution utilizing open-systems technology will maximize reuse and broaden market acceptance.

As noted above, decision support either can be tightly coupled with a host clinical-information system, in the form of embedded in-line code, or can be implemented as a more loosely coupled second system that operates as an adjunct to the primary clinical-care system. An example of in-line code is embedded code within an order-entry system that provides medication dose-adjustment advice during order-entry workflow; an example of a loosely coupled second system is a system or program that monitors events in order to generate alerts to providers about worsening laboratory values.

Clinical Decision Support Successes and Obstacles

Several institutions have developed their own implementations of event-based CDSS; these programs perform active monitoring as a result of the integration of decision support with medical-record systems. Primary among these systems are the Health Evaluation through Logical Processing (HELP) system from LDS Hospital in Salt Lake City,[1] the Regenstrief Medical Record System (RMRS) from the Regenstrief Institute for Healthcare in Indianapolis,[2 3] a decision-support system at Columbia-Presbyterian Medical Center (CPMC),[4] and the Brigham Integrated Computing System (BICS) at Brigham and Women's Hospital in Boston.[5] These efforts have demonstrated cost savings, an improved quality of care, and the capability of changing the behavior of clinicians, although additional metrics need to be developed. All have used proprietary databases, locally built decision-support servers, and different forms of controlled vocabularies and data dictionaries. These systems have been in routine use in their home institutions since the early 1980s. A commercial version of HELP is being actively marketed and deployed, and other vendor systems that employ the ideas in these pioneering systems have been developed and are now starting to be deployed in increasing numbers.

Obstacles to the widespread deployment of CDSS remain. First, the healthcare industry has a major investment in a variety of "proven" legacy information systems that are costly and difficult to replace. These systems often were not designed to interoperate. System integration is feasible through interface engines and standards such as HL7 (Health Level Seven), but the cost is still significant. A second obstacle is the brittle nature of legacy system code; it is difficult to intervene at the appropriate part of the workflow in order to make CDSS techniques palatable. Third, insufficient availability and poor encoding of clinical data preclude the application of sophisticated CDSS techniques. The remaining sections of this paper address a fourth major obstacle to the wide deployment of CDSS—the lack of standards for representation of both healthcare data and clinical logic. The industry is slowly making progress with regard to these obstacles, but the impact of the "mission-critical" setting for healthcare delivery and its associated information systems makes healthcare a conservative, risk-averse environment when it comes to rapid change.

Emerging Standards

Work in standards development for CDSS addresses a variety of needs. The three primary areas are: representation of clinical logic and guidelines to enhance shareability, convergence of a clinical data model to support encoded logic, and identification and standardization of the interfaces between a CDSS and its host environment.

There are two aspects of the standardization of guidelines to leverage for CDSS: guideline content standards and guideline structure standards. Several organizations have developed and disseminated standards for guideline content that are gaining acceptance, and in addition there are locally developed guidelines. These include the indicators of the Joint Commission on Accreditation of Health Care Organizations for assessing provider performance and the Health Plan Employer Data and Information Set quality performance measures. Other national, regional, and professional associations such as the American Medical Association, the American College of Physicians, and the federal Agency for Health Care Policy and Research at the Public Health Service have developed practice guidelines. Individual provider institutions such as CPMC and Massachusetts General Hospital are also devising their own clinical guidelines. Finally, other private organizations have developed and marketed practice guidelines, such as Health Risk Management's Institute for Healthcare Quality, Value Health Sciences, and Milliman & Robertson, Inc.[6]

In the area of standardization of guideline structure, work is being pursued both within established standards bodies such as the American Society for Testing and Materials (ASTM) and HL7 and in the academic medical informatics community, notably within the InterMed collaboration among Columbia, Harvard, and Stanford universities. Efforts to apply a reference clinical-information model to decision support are also being made within HL7, which is an American National Standards Institute (ANSI)-accredited standards body dedicated to information exchange among healthcare systems. Finally, the development of standard interfaces for CDSS had been undertaken by both HL7 and the CORBAmed Domain Task Force of the Object Management Group (OMG).

Arden Syntax Medical-Logic Modules. A standardized representation for medical logic and guidelines is one enabler for building repeatable decision-support systems. The Arden Syntax for knowledge representation is a balloted and internationally deployed standard that was created with the goal of allowing users to create and share pieces of medical knowledge in a form that can be implemented by computer systems. The Arden Syntax was developed under the auspices of the E31.15 subcommittee (Health Knowledge Representation) of the ASTM, which is an ANSI-approved standards-development organization (SDO). The standard was developed as E1460-92, the Standard Specification for Defining and Sharing Modular Health Knowledge Bases, but is generally referred to simply as the Arden Syntax. Because of a confluence of complementary activities within other standards groups, the Arden Syntax has come under the HL7 umbrella, another ANSI SDO, and is now maintained within the Clinical Decision Support Technical Committee of HL7.

The Arden Syntax was developed primarily to address the need for "data-driven" decision support, which means that logic rules are invoked as a result of changes to the patient data in a clinical system. The syntax was based on the experiences of pioneer homegrown CDSS, in particular the HELP system and the RMRS/CARE system. Its primary objective is to enable sharing of medical knowledge by providing a standard language for clinical decision rules. Clinical rules are encoded as medical-logic modules (MLMs). Each MLM contains the knowledge sufficient for making a single clinical decision. MLMs are designed to function independently but can also be devised to call one another, as subroutines do.

Each MLM has three main sections: maintenance, library, and knowledge. Each of these sections is made up of several slots that contain further information. The maintenance and library sections are used primarily to facilitate maintenance of the rule knowledge base. The main part of an MLM is in the knowledge section. The required patient data and the coupling of rule variables to the institution-specific knowledge bases are specified in the data slot. The evoke slot defines what event triggers this piece of medical logic, and the logic slot contains the actual procedural logic that should be performed when the rule is triggered. The action slot specifies what should happen when the logic in the logic slot evaluates to true. Additional aspects of the rule definition are message destination and priority and urgency ratings. Temporal relations are a central feature of the Arden Syntax because they play a distinct and important role in clinical reasoning. Every data value is associated with a primary time, which is the medically relevant time for that data value. For example, for a laboratory result the primary time is generally the time the specimen was drawn, and the time of a laboratory-order event is the time the order was actually placed. The syntax also contains numerous powerful constructs for specifying time constraints such as within, preceding, following, same day as, before, and after, and methods for specifying repeating events at specified cycles, scheduled events, or delayed events. Hripcsak and others give a comprehensive description of the Arden Syntax and of the motivation for it.[7] A website with extensive information and sample rules is at www.cpmc.columbia.edu/ resources/arden. A sample MLM illustrating the features discussed is shown in Exhibit 1.

MLMs are commonly used to represent alerts and reminders in clinical-information systems. The additional infrastructure required for implementation includes several software tools. The basic tools are: an MLM authoring tool with configuration-management capability, an Arden Syntax compiler or translator, a decision-support engine to actually execute the rule logic, and trigger, query, and notification handlers. Unfortunately, at the present time, there are few commercial tools and components in these areas. Development of componented solutions by vendors for the required Arden Syntax infrastructure will go a long way in furthering adoption and widespread implementation of the standard. In addition, because Arden specifies neither a data model nor an architecture, it is still difficult to implement shared rules across implementations without significant changes and testing. Further progress within other standards bodies toward developing clinical vocabularies and reference-information models may reduce this obstacle and facilitate more widespread deployment of Arden Syntax–based CDSS.

A number of vendors of clinical-information systems have implemented CDSS based on the Arden Syntax, including HealthVision, IBM, SMS, and 3M. These implementations include generally available Arden Syntax–based products and live projects in customer healthcare institutions. Other vendors, such as Cerner and HBOC, have Arden Syntax projects either in a planning phase

Exhibit 1. Example of an Arden Syntax Rule

Maintenance:
>   title: Screen for hypokalemia with digoxin therapy;;
>   filename: hypokalemia_and_digoxin;;
>   version: 1.06;;
>   institution: Columbia-Presbyterian Medical Center;;
>   author: George Hripcsak, M.D. (hripcsa@cuccis.columbia.edu);;
>   date: 1993-09-17;;
>   validation: production;;

Library:
>   purpose: Warn provider of hypokalemia in setting of digoxin therapy;
>   explanation: Whenever a serum or whole blood potassium value is stored, check
>   for hypokalemia (< 3.3).;;
>   keywords: hypokalemia; digoxin; arrhythmia ;;
>   citations: 1.. NEJM 1991;324:424-8.;;
>   links: CTIM-1.14.5;;

Knowledge:
>   type: data-driven;;
>   data: K := read last {serum potassium value} where it occurred before now;;
>   priority: 50;;
>   evoke: potassium_storage;;
>   logic: if K >= 3.3 then conclude false; endif;;
>   action: write îThis patient has hypokalemia in the setting of digoxin therapy....î;;

End:

---

or under development. In addition to these commercial applications, a number of academic institutions use Arden Syntax in their CDSS.

Guideline Interchange Format. Although successful implementations of the Arden Syntax exist, the syntax is limited with regard to the representation of complex, multipart guidelines and protocols for care. Although many time-related operators are supported within the logic of a single MLM, it is generally difficult to coordinate multiple medical-logic modules in the complicated temporal way necessary to represent lengthy clinical guidelines. In order for these increasingly important guidelines to be shared by institutions in media other than text, new representations must be explored. The Guideline Interchange Format (GLIF) is being developed for this purpose by the InterMed Collaboratory, which is a partnership of investigators from Columbia, Harvard, and Stanford universities.[8]

GLIF resulted from the analysis of four existing guideline systems: Arden Syntax–based medical-logic modules from Columbia, Guided Entry of Data Elements-Clinical Medicine at Brigham and Women's Hospital, Modeling Better Treatment Advice at Massachusetts General Hospital, and EON at Stanford. Features of a GLIF guideline object include a guideline intention, eligibility criteria, and guideline steps. In order to represent the needed temporal logic, guideline steps may be action steps, conditional steps, branch steps, and synchronization steps. The evaluation of the resulting guideline syntax found it to be capable of expressing guidelines from all participants in the collaboration, although it is possible to express the same guideline in many ways. The ability to share GLIF-encoded guidelines is limited by a lack of a standard clinical-data model and vocabulary, which is also the prime obstacle to the shareability of the Arden Syntax.

The acceptance of guideline-standardization approaches such as the Arden Syntax and GLIF will play a role in facilitating repeatable decision-support implementations within the client-server component-based computing paradigm.

HL7 and the Clinical Decision Support Technical Committee. In April 1996 a special-interest group (SIG) on decision support was formed within HL7. Two projects have been pursued within this working group: near-real-time alerts and data warehousing. In August 1998, the SIG was broken into two technical committees (TCs) to address the obviously different needs of the projects: the CDSS TC and the Data Warehousing TC. The ASTM Arden Syntax subcommittee has been absorbed into the CDSS TC because the Arden Syntax is used within decision-support systems and because its shareability and standardization goals strongly overlap with the concerns of the HL7 group. The CDSS TC has focused on identifying the common blocks of functionality within CDSS design. The primary architectural pieces of a CDSS that may need to exchange information have been identified as the event source, trigger or dispatcher, clinical data sources, logic engine, notifier, destination, acknowledger, and alert log. There may be more than one of each of these components. Even though the patterns of communications differ in constituent systems, the components that require communication and their general functions are shared by all examined constituent systems or designs. The CDSS TC is continuing to flesh out the components further in terms of communication needs via use cases.

The CDSS TC is also addressing the lack of standardization of data access within CDSS rules or guidelines. For example, one of the major challenges in using and sharing Arden Syntax rules is the lack of standard ways to refer to the clinical data utilized within the rule logic. Because every database in a host system is different, and there is no standard data model or clinical terminology, the parts of the rules that refer to the data must be translated for or mapped on the local data model and local terminology. The Arden Syntax designers recognized this problem and adopted a neutral position by isolating the institution-dependent parts of the rule within "curly brackets" (sometimes also referred to as "curly braces") in the DATA section of the rules. Thus a buffer is provided between the nonstandardized clinical-information system and the standardized CDSS logic. This "deferring" of the data-access dilemma has been dubbed the "curly-brackets" problem. Members of the HL7 CDSS TC (formerly of ASTM) have done some work on outlining the components needed for a generalized solution. The major components are: a standard-reference data model, a standard query language that refers to this model, and standard-reference clinical vocabularies for all clinical data. Clearly developing these components is a large task, but emerging work within HL7 on the Reference Information Model and the forecasted adoption of comprehensive and useable clinical terminologies such as Systematized Nomenclature of Human Medicine-Reference Terminology, READ, and Logical Observation Identifier Names and Codes are hopeful indicators of convergence. In addition, work on the standardization of principles—and, to some extent, content—of clinical vocabularies is being undertaken by the HL7 Vocabulary Technical Committee.

CORBAmed Healthcare Data Interpretation Facility. The OMG (www.omg.org) has established a number of vertical domain task forces to specify requirements for object interfaces, one of which is the CORBAmed Domain Task Force. Within CORBAmed, a work group was established to solicit and develop specifications for CDSS. The goal of the specifications is the eventual adoption of vendor-neutral common interfaces that may improve the quality of care and reduce costs by utilizing CORBA (standard) technologies for the interoperability of systems, applications, and instruments that detect, transmit, store, and display the medical information used in CDSS and thus the standardization of interfaces for related healthcare objects.[9][10] To that end, in June 1997, the OMG issued a request for information that could be used to develop the requirements for the request for proposals (RFP) to vendors.

The RFP, entitled "Healthcare Data Interpretation Facility" (HDIF), was issued in March 1998. This name was chosen in order to differentiate the financial and clinical uses of the term *decision-support system*. Submitted proposals were to address (1) the accommodation of different intelligent transforms of clinical data, (2) the easy integration of intelligent systems into existing healthcare information systems, and (3) the common interfaces for performing intelligent transforms of healthcare data distributed across disparate healthcare-data domains. The requirements for a specification of a standardized HDIF include interfaces that can serve and encapsulations for heterogenous "data-transform" techniques that might be used in healthcare-data interpretation, such as a set of rules, a neural network, fuzzy-logic techniques, or statistical algorithms. Additional specifications include the ability to chain inputs and outputs required for multiple transforms, the ability to provide references or explanations of the behavior of transforms, specification of the (preferably public) clinical vocabularies utilized, and alignment with other work emerging from other CORBAmed work groups: Clinical Observations Access Service, Lexicon Query Services, and Patient Identification Services. The mechanisms for the notification (alerts, warnings) and presentation were noted clearly to be outside the scope of this RFP. Responses to the RFP are scheduled to be received, reviewed, and approved during the first part of 1999.

Conclusion

Clinical-information systems that are enhanced with CDSS capabilities are finally beginning to emerge in vendor systems. In order to facilitate repeatable, reusable, and easily modified systems, standards are needed. Although locally based efforts have been well publicized for many years, several viable forces in the standards and vendor communities are beginning to converge and are likely to result in faster progress. Events such as the absorption of the Arden Syntax committee into the HL7 Decision Support TC, increased collaboration between HL7 and CORBAmed, and aggressive activities within HL7's Vocabulary TC will encourage further standardization efforts for CDSS. In addition, academic groups, such as the InterMed group working on GLIF and academic medical informatics department, should be encouraged to channel their work and requirements through the existing standards efforts to facilitate progress and increase synergy. Standards are likely to emerge in the areas of vocabulary and software components.

References

1. Pryor, T. A., Gardner, R. M., Clayton, P. D., and Warner, H. R., Jr. "The HELP System." In B. I. Blum (ed.), *Information Systems for Patient Care*. New York: Springer-Verlag, 1984.
2. McDonald, C. J. *Action-Oriented Decisions in Ambulatory Medicine*. St. Louis, Mo.: Mosby-Year Book, 1981.
3. McDonald, C. J., Tierney, W. M., Martin, D. K., and Overhage, J. M. "The Regenstrief Medical Record System: 20 Years of Experience in Hospitals, Clinics and Neighborhood Health Centers." *MD Computing,* 1992, *9* (4), 206–217.
4. Hripcsak, G., Cimino, J., Johnson, S., and Clayton, P. "The Columbia-Presbyterian Medical Center Decision-Support System as a Model for Implementing the Arden Syntax." In *Proceedings of 15th SCAMC.* New York: McGraw-Hill, 1991.
5. Glaser, J., and Kuperman, G. J. "Impact of Information Events on Medical Care." *Proceedings of the Healthcare Information Management Systems Society Conference,* 1996, *2,* 2–9.
6. Blair, J. S. "An Overview of Health Care Information Standards." *Proceedings of the Healthcare Information and Management Systems Society,* 1996, pp. 203–212.
7. Hripcsak, G., and others. "Rationale for the Arden Syntax." *Computers and Biomedical Research,* 1994, *27* (4), 291–324.
8. Ohno-Machado, L., and others. "The GuideLine Interchange Format: A Model for Representing Guidelines." *Journal of the American Medical Informatics Association,* July/August 1998, *5* (4), 357–372.
9. *CORBAmed RFI 3: Clinical Decision Support, Object Management Group.* OMG Document: corbamed/97-06-05. New Mexico: Object Management Group, June 1997.
10. *CORBAmed Request for Proposal: Healthcare Data Interpretation Facility.* OMG Document: corbamed/98-03-29. New Mexico: Object Management Group, March 1998.

About the Author

Carol A. Broverman, Ph.D., is senior informatics specialist at Oceania, in Redwood City, California.

Differential Diagnosis

Eta S. Berner, Ed.D.

Diagnostic decision-support systems (DDSS), as the name implies, are designed to assist a clinician with the process of diagnosis. Key words in that definition are *assist, process,* and *diagnosis.* These systems do not make the diagnosis for the clinician but provide a variety of functions that can assist the user in arriving at a diagnosis. As Miller and Geissbuhler describe, diagnosis is not simply getting an answer; it is a process that includes a variety of subprocesses. As described by Miller and Geissbuhler and others, this process includes gathering appropriate information from the patient, interpreting that information properly, generating diagnostic hypotheses, and gathering additional information to assist in evaluating and refining these hypotheses.[1][2][3][4]

Some "diagnostic" systems focus on the identification of abnormalities in narrow clinical domains. For instance, computer programs assist in the interpretation of mammograms and pap smears by alerting the radiologist or cytotechnologist to potentially cancerous tissue changes that might have been overlooked.[5][6] Also, most electrocardiographic systems have a module that generates interpretations of the electrocardiograph (ECG) patterns.[7] All these systems provide suggestions that the clinician must interpret, but the clinician makes the final determination as to whether abnormalities are present.

The systems that assist with differential diagnosis, however, involve the integration of many types of data or evidence, a method to evaluate the strength of the evidence using a knowledge base of rules or associative linkages, and they infer likely diagnoses given the evidence and the knowledge-base model. Examples of these systems are Quick Medical Reference (QMR), originally developed at the University of Pittsburgh and currently commercially available through First DataBank; DXplain, developed at and available via the web from Massachusetts General Hospital; Iliad, originally developed by Applied Medical Informatics at the University of Utah and currently available from A.D.A.M. Internet Health; and Problem-Knowledge Coupler, available from PKC Corporation. DDSS have also been developed for differential diagnosis in subspecialty areas.

The broad-based systems designed to assist with differential diagnosis will be discussed here. This article (1) gives a brief description of the evolution of DDSS, (2) discusses the factors that must be addressed for these systems to be widely implemented, (3) describes some of the functions of the systems, (4) summarizes the data on the evaluation of system accuracy and impact, and (5) identifies issues to be addressed in the future with regard to the implementation of DDSS. Although some aspects of specific systems may be used as illustrations, the article is not a comprehensive review of any one of the systems but rather provides an overview of the type of functionality and performance that can be expected from systems that provide decision support for differential diagnosis.

Historical Overview of Diagnostic Decision Support Systems

Research began on prototypes for many of the DDSS that are commercially available today over 25 years ago. Many of these early systems, as Miller discusses in an excellent review of the history of these programs, were intended as an application of artificial intelligence–based expert-system methodology to the medical domain.[8] Although some of the programs were broad-based diagnostic systems (for example, Internist-1 and the pediatric version of Meditel),[9][10] many of the early systems were targeted at narrow problem areas, such as infectious diseases,[11] determination of acid-base status,[12] or evaluation of the acute abdomen.[13]

The 1980s brought further developments of these expert systems and the development of new broad-based systems (Meditel for adults, Iliad, and DXplain).[14][15][16] However, during this period, it became apparent to many systems developers that, instead of trying to develop an expert system to provide a differential diagnosis, it would be more fruitful to use the extensive information in the knowledge bases of these systems to develop a more interactive system that could be used to support physician diagnostic exploration.[17] For example, QMR was developed using the structure and content of the Internist-1 knowledge base but with a more interactive user interface, increased functionality, and an intent to focus on the decision-support rather than the expert-system mode.[18] QMR, Meditel, Iliad, DXplain, and Problem-Knowledge Coupler, while using different knowledge bases and different algorithms, all have a similar intent— to compile extant knowledge so that it can be applied to patient-specific information to assist the clinician with the development of a differential diagnosis.

Standards and Methods for Implementing Diagnostic Decision Support Systems

Although some of the functions of these DDSS are similar, there are no agreed-on standards for knowledge-base models, inference algorithms, user interface, or mode of user interaction. All of the major DDSS referred to above take as input a given patient's signs and symptoms (and some also take laboratory data) as input and produce a list of possible diagnoses. Some of the systems allow the input of "normal" findings, while others accept only abnormal patient data. These data must be entered using the controlled vocabulary of the system, which is matched to the information in the knowledge base. The knowledge bases of the various systems contain information on the degree of association of various signs and symptoms with hundreds, and for some systems thousands, of diseases. The knowledge in the systems usually is based on data from the medical literature, experts, or actual patients (or some combination of these sources). Various inference algorithms are used (depending on the particular DDSS) to combine the patient's findings (signs, symptoms) with the disease information in the knowledge base in order to produce a list of diagnostic possibilities, ranked in order of likelihood. Some systems base their algorithms on Bayesian models, while others use ad hoc quasi-probabilistic scoring schemes that take into account disease prevalence and the strength of the association of the signs and symptoms with each disease.[19] Problem-Knowledge Coupler uses a combinatorial algorithm that does not include probabilistic information. Currently, the predominant mode of data entry for these systems is for the user to enter the patient's data. Although Problem-Knowledge Coupler is designed for nonphysician data entry, the other systems assume that a physician or similarly qualified health professional will provide the patient data for the system. DXplain is available on the web from the Massachusetts General Hospital server; QMR can be used stand-alone or via an intranet; and Iliad and Problem-Knowledge Coupler are stand-alone programs.

Critical Functionality of Diagnostic Decision Support Systems

The user of these systems needs to understand the assumptions under which the systems operate. The DDSS are designed to provide suggestions about differential diagnosis, not to determine the patient's definitive diagnosis. The lists provided are often lengthy, and the patient's actual diagnosis may not always be at the top of the list. The actual diagnosis may be farther down on the list either because the disease is unusual and the more common diseases are likely to be listed first or because the patient has an unusual case presentation with few of the classic findings for the disease. In any case, the programs assume that a competent physician, who may have more information about the patient than was able to be entered into the system, will sort through the suggestions and ignore those that are not helpful.

System performance can be sensitive to the data that are entered. The clinician needs to enter as much pertinent data as are available. For most of the systems the clinician user must both identify pertinent data and also select the appropriate DDSS term from the controlled system vocabulary. Therefore, errors can arise from the omission of pertinent data and from inputting incorrect terms. Further, in an effort to save time, the physician may omit important data. These errors can cause the DDSS to perform suboptimally. Problem-Knowledge Coupler addresses this problem by having all patients answer the same lengthy set of questions related to the chief complaint. To conserve physician time, a nonphysician collects these data and provides the physician with the system's analysis of the data. However, because Problem-Knowledge Coupler does not use probabilistic information to eliminate unlikely diseases, the more findings that are entered, the longer the list of potential diagnoses might be. Automating the process of initial data entry not only may reduce the data entry time but also may improve system performance.

It is also assumed that these programs do not function statically, in what has been termed the "Greek oracle" mode, where the main role of the user is to enter patient data and let the system analyze it.[17] The systems are designed for extensive user interaction. In addition to generating diagnostic suggestions, these programs may have other ways of assisting the clinician. They can function as an electronic textbook so that the clinician can view the findings associated with given diseases or can look at relevant references. The systems can also suggest additional data that could be gathered to work up a particular finding or to rule in or rule out a particular diagnosis. One of the important functions is to provide an explanation of why a particular diagnosis was suggested by the system or why a diagnosis that the clinician was thinking of was not generated by the DDSS. For instance, if a clinician wanted to find out why QMR suggested a particular diagnosis for a patient, she could have QMR "critique" that diagnosis. The critique function lists the patient's symptoms that indicate a given disease and identifies which of the patient's signs and symptoms are not associated with the particular disease and which key features in the disease are not present in the particular patient. The system also suggests the gathering of additional data that might confirm the diagnosis. The other DDSS have similar functions. An illustration of how this function looks on DXplain can be seen in a demonstration of DXplain at www.lcs.mgh.harvard.edu/dxpdemo/frame26.htm.

The clinician can also find out whether a disease is even in the system's knowledge base; its absence might be the main reason it was not suggested. Although early research into physician's attitudes toward computer-assisted diagnosis emphasized that physicians felt that the ability of the system to explain its "reasoning" was extremely important,[20] a more recent study has shown that physicians who have purchased the systems do not always seek that explanation.[21] Perhaps knowing that the explanation is available is an important factor in deciding to purchase the system but is less important once the system is in use. Also, the electronic-textbook features can also be thought of as providing some explanation of the reasoning, and system users may be more comfortable with these features than with the more sophisticated critiquing functions.[21] It is also possible that many cases do not require the use of the more sophisticated functions or that physicians do not have the time for extensive interaction. However, it is also possible that the clinicians do not know how to use the full range of features available in these systems, which raises the question of user training.

Although all systems have a user manual or online help functions (or both), there is debate about whether these systems should be totally intuitive or whether the user needs additional training to know how to use them properly. At the very least the user needs to understand the variety of features that are available, how to use them, and how to interpret their output. In addition, since the DDSS have a controlled vocabulary for finding description and disease nomenclature, the user may need some experience with the system to understand how various terms are used. Also, the user will need practice in interacting with the system, using various functions, or adding more data in order to understand how to refine the suggestions that are initially produced.

Impact of Diagnostic Decision Support Systems

Although DDSS have been systematically studied, there have been few controlled trials of the systems in clinical practice situations[22]. Results of evaluations of the systems themselves (rather than of how they are used) have been mixed[23], but research has shown that these systems include the correct diagnosis in their list of suggestions at least half the time,[24] that physicians perceive them as helpful,[25] and that physicians' diagnoses can be improved.[26 27] Some studies have suggested that these systems can also be useful in an educational setting—for instance, for residents in training.[28 29] Iliad, in fact, was originally developed as an educational tool, and most of the other systems have been used to educate physicians, nurses, and other health professionals.[30]

The ECG-interpretation programs mentioned earlier have had similar evaluations, but they, unlike the differential-diagnosis programs, were able to be easily incorporated into the routine ECG output.[31] Of course, this incorporation has mainly involved printing the suggestions on the ECG tracings, and it is not known to what extent that information is routinely used by the clinicians who have to interpret the tracings. Studies have shown that the ECG-interpretation suggestions can affect physicians' diagnoses.[32 33]but also that physicians vary in how accurate they perceive these suggestions to be.[34] One of the main differences between the ECG programs and the other DDSS is that the input data for the ECG programs are automated and do not need physician interpretation, while the DDSS programs require separate clinical-data selection, interpretation, and entry. Without automated data entry it is likely that the potential of these systems will not be fully realized.

Future Trends

Although some changes may be made in the inference algorithms of the systems, the more likely trends are (1) linking the systems to a computer-based patient record (CPR) so that initial data entry can be automated,

(2) developing a system for regular updating and maintenance of the knowledge bases, and (3) developing training procedures so that users will interact properly with the DDSS. The user interfaces will probably also become more standardized.

As CPR systems develop and come into routine use, the opportunities to provide links to a DDSS will increase.[35] Such links will allow the initial patient data to be obtained automatically, which not only could make data entry more efficient but may make it more accurate as well. Some efforts are already under way, such as the Wizorder project at Vanderbilt University.[36] The variability in clinical vocabulary is still problematic, both for capturing the clinical data in a CPR and for translating that data for input into a DDSS. Most of the DDSS have some sort of synonym dictionary that might be able to be expanded to accommodate a broader range of terms. In addition, the controlled vocabulary from some of the DDSS is now in the National Library of Medicine's Unified Medical Language System (UMLS), which may help that mapping process, especially for any CPR systems that use UMLS to link controlled vocabularies as part of a broader system design.[37]

Maintenance and upgrading of the knowledge base continues to be an issue that must be addressed. The knowledge bases of all the systems need review and updating, and the DDSS with the smaller knowledge bases need to increase their coverage. The knowledge-acquisition process is time-consuming; however, technological developments may make that process easier. Several knowledge-engineering tools have been developed that ensure consistency between the existing knowledge bases and new diseases and findings that are added.[38] As web interfaces become more prevalent, other systems may develop an easier way for distributing the updated information, as DXplain has already. In addition, once DDSS are linked to a CPR, the patient data collected could also be used to refine the DDSS knowledge base and make it more sensitive to local conditions. However, given that there are often unexplained variations in practice styles within small geographic areas,[39] using local data could make the DDSS more biased if it incorporates unusual diagnostic strategies, practice styles, or patient populations.

Finally, if these systems come into routine use, some systematic training will likely accompany them. Proper training in use of the system may be able to compensate for limitations in the number of diseases in the knowledge bases and for lack of specificity in the diagnostic suggestions.

Don Tapscott, in his book *Growing Up Digital*,[40] predicts that as the children and teenagers of today enter the workforce, they will expect to use computers routinely in all their activities. Although today few of the differential-diagnosis systems are in routine use, as the technology matures and as Tapscott's "net generation" enters clinical practice, these types of decision-support systems will likely become a routine part of the clinician's armamentarium.

References

1. Miller, R. A., and Geissbuhler, A. "Clinical Decision Support Systems—An Overview." In E. S. Berner (ed.), *Clinical Decision Support Systems: Theory and Practice.* New York: Springer-Verlag, 1998.
2. Elstein, A. S., Shulman, L. S., and Sprafka, S. A. *Medical Problem Solving: An Analysis of Clinical Reasoning.* Cambridge, Mass.: Harvard University Press, 1978.
3. Eddy, D. M., and Clanton, C. H. "The Art of Diagnosis: Solving the Clinicopathological Exercise." *New England Journal of Medicine,* 1982, *306,* 1493–1499.
4. Kassirer, J. P. "Teaching Clinical Medicine by Iterative Hypothesis Testing. Let's Preach What We Practice." *New England Journal of Medicine,* 1983, *309,* 921–923.
5. Rothenberg, L. N. "Mammography Instrumentation: Recent Developments." *Medical Progress Through Technology,* 1993, *19,* 1–6.
6. Mango, L. J. "Computer-Assisted Cervical Cancer Screening Using Neural Networks." *Cancer Letters,* 1994, *77,* 155–162.
7. Drazen, E., Mann, N., Borun, R., Laks, M., and Bersen, A. "Survey of Computer-Assisted Electrocardiography in the United States." *Journal of Electrocardiology,* 1988 (supplement), S98–S104.
8. Miller, R. A. "Medical Diagnostic Decision Support Systems—Past, Present, and Future: A Threaded Bibliography and Commentary." *Journal of the American Medical Informatics Association,* 1994, *1,* 8–27.
9. Miller, R. A., Pople, H. E., Jr., and Myers, J. D. "Internist-1, an Experimental Computer-Based Diagnostic Consultant for General Internal Medicine." *New England Journal of Medicine,* 1982, *307* (8), 468–476.
10. Barness, L. A., Tunnessen, W. W., Jr., Worley, W. E., Simmons, T. L., and Ringe, T.B.K., Jr. "Computer-Assisted Diagnosis in Pediatrics." *American Journal of Diseases in Children,* 1974, *127,* 852–858.
11. Shortliffe, E. H. *Computer-Based Medical Consultations: MYCIN.* Artificial Intelligence Series. New York: Elsevier, 1976.
12. Bleich, H. L. "Computer Evaluation of the Acid-Base Disorders." *Journal of Clinical Investigation,* 1969, *48,* 1689–1696.
13. de Dombal, F. T. "Computer-Aided Diagnosis and Decision Making in the Acute Abdomen." *Journal of the Royal College of Physicians,* 1975, *9,* 211–218.
14. Waxman, H. S., and Worley, W. E. "Computer-Assisted Adult Medical Diagnosis: Subject Review and Evaluation of a New Microcomputer-Based System." *Medicine,* 1990, *69,* 125–136.
15. Warner, H. R., Jr. "Iliad: Moving Medical Decision-Making into New Frontiers." *Methods of Information in Medicine,* 1989, *28* (4), 370–372.
16. Barnett, G. O., Cimino, J. J., Hupp, J. A., and Hoffer, E. P. "DXplain: An Evolving Diagnostic Decision-Support System." *Journal of the American Medical Association,* 1987, *258* (1), 67–74.
17. Miller, R. A., and Masarie, F. E., Jr. "The Demise of the 'Greek Oracle' Model for Medical Diagnostic Systems." *Methods of Information in Medicine,* 1990, *29,* 1–2.
18. Miller, R. A., McNeil, M., Challinor, S., Masarie, F. E., Jr., and Myers, J. D. "The Internist-1/Quick Medical Reference Project—Status Report. *Western Journal of Medicine,* 1986, *145,* 816–822.
19. Spooner, A. S. "Mathematical Foundations of Decision Support Systems." In E. S. Berner (ed.), *Clinical Decision Support Systems: Theory and Practice.* New York: Springer-Verlag, 1998.
20. Teach, R. L., and Shortliffe, E. H. "An Analysis of Physician Attitudes Regarding Computer-Based Clinical Consultation Systems." *Computers and Biomedical Research,* 1981, *14,* 542–558.

21. Berner, E. S., and Maisiak, R. S. "Physician Use of Interactive Functions in Diagnostic Decision Support Systems." *Proceedings, AMIA Fall Symposium,* 1997, p. 842.

22. Hunt, D. L., Haynes, R. B., Hanna, S. E., and Smith, K. "Effects of Computer-Based Clinical Decision Support Systems on Physician Performance and Patient Outcomes. A Systematic Review." *Journal of the American Medical Association,* 1998, *280* (15), 1339–1346.

23. Berner, E. S. "Testing System Accuracy." In E. S. Berner (ed.), *Clinical Decision Support Systems: Theory and Practice.* New York: Springer-Verlag, 1998.

24. Berner, E. S., and others, "Performance of Four Computer-Based Diagnostic Systems." *New England Journal of Medicine,* 1994, *330* (25), 1792–1796.

25. Berner, E. S., and Maisiak, R. S. "Factors Affecting Physician Evaluation of Diagnostic Decision Support Systems." Paper presented at the Spring Congress, American Medical Informatics Association, Philadelphia, May 1998.

26. Berner, E. S., Maisiak, R. S., Cobbs, C. G., and Taunton, O. D. "Effects of a Decision Support System on Physician Diagnostic Performance." Unpublished paper.

27. Elstein, A. S., Friedman, C. P., Wolf, F. M., Murphy, G. C., Franz, T. M., Heckerling, P. S., Fine, P. L., Miller, T. M., and Miller, J. "Enhancement of Diagnostic Reasoning by a Computer-Based Decision Support System." *Medical Decision Making,* 1998, *18,* 458.

28. Bankowitz, R. A., McNeil, M. A., Challinor, S. M., Parker, R. C., Kapoor, W. N., and Miller, R. A. "A Computer-Assisted Medical Diagnostic Consultation Service: Implementation and Prospective Evaluation of a Prototype." *Annals of Internal Medicine,* 1989, *110* (10), 824–832.

29. Bacchus, C. M., Quinton, C., O'Rourke, K., Detsky, A. S. "A Randomized Crossover Trial of Quick Medical Reference (QMR) as a Teaching Tool for Medical Interns." *Journal of General Internal Medicine,* 1994, *9,* 616–621.

30. Lincoln, M. J. "Medical Education Applications." In E. S. Berner (ed.), *Clinical Decision Support Systems: Theory and Practice.* New York: Springer-Verlag, 1998.

31. Willems, J. L., and others, "The Diagnostic Performance of Computer Programs for the Interpretation of Electrocardiograms." *New England Journal of Medicine,* 1991, 325 (25), 1767–1773.

32. Wooley, D., Henck, M., and Luck, J. "Comparison of Electrocardiogram Interpretations by Family Physicians, a Computer, and a Cardiology Service." *Journal of Family Practice,* 1992, *34,* 428–432.

33. Hillson, S. D., Connelly, D. P., and Liu, Y. "The Effects of Computer-Assisted Electrocardiographic Interpretation on Physicians' Diagnostic Decisions." *Medical Decision Making,* 1995, *15,* 107–112.

34. Berner, E. S., Kennedy, J. I., Blackwell, G., and Box, J. B. "Use of Computer-Generated ECG Reports by Residents and Faculty." In *Proceedings of the Nineteenth Annual Symposium of Computer Applications in Medical Care.* Philadelphia: Hanley & Belfus, 1995.

35. Dick, R. S., Steen, E. B., and Detmer, D. E. *The Computer-Based Patient Record: An Essential Technology for Health Care.* (Rev. ed.) Washington, D.C.: National Academy Press, 1997.

36. Geissbuhler, A., and Miller, R. A. "A New Approach to the Implementation of Direct Care-Provider Order Entry." *Proceedings, AMIA Fall Symposium,* 1996, pp. 689–693.

37. Humphreys, B. L., Lindberg, D.A.B., Schoolman, H. M., and Barnett, G. O. "The Unified Medical Language System: An Informatics Research Collaboration." *Journal of the American Medical Informatics Association,* 1998, *5,* 1–11.

38. Giuse, D. A., Giuse, N. B., and Miller, R. A. "Consistency Enforcement in Medical Knowledge Base Construction." *Artificial Intelligence in Medicine,* 1993, *5,* 245–252.

39. Wennberg, D. E., Kellett, M. A., Dickens, J. D., Malenka, D. J., Keilson, L. M., and Keller, R. B. "The Association Between Local Diagnostic Testing Intensity and Invasive Cardiac Procedures." *Journal of the American Medical Association,* 1996, *275,* 1161–1164.

40. Tapscott, D. *Growing Up Digital.* New York: McGraw-Hill, 1998.

About the Author

Eta S. Berner, Ed.D., is professor in the Department of Health Services Administration, School of Health Related Professions, University of Alabama at Birmingham. She teaches in the Master of Science of Health Informatics Program.

Medication-Management Issues at the Point of Care

John Poikonen, R.Ph.; John M. Leventhal, M.D.

In hospitals and in the outpatient environment, drug budgets are exploding because of the overuse of expensive drugs with dubious therapeutic advantage over older, less expensive alternatives and because new therapeutic agents are being approved at record rates. Adverse drug events are now the fourth leading cause of death in the United States,[1] the equivalent of a commercial plane crash every day. It is easy to see why many healthcare organizations and institutions target drug therapy as one of the first areas in which to implement decision-support services.

Computerized decision support via pharmacy order entry at the point of dispensing has been in practice for many years. Given the high rates of adverse drug reactions and prescribing errors, pharmacists using these systems have not been very successful in providing good clinical decision support. The reasons include the disconnect of time and data from the point of care to the point of dispensing. Online prescriber order entry would enable decision-support systems to provide potentially critical information close to the moment of decision making. Shifting order entry and clinical decision support to the point of care offers tremendous benefits and challenges. This discussion will draw on the experience of pharmacy-based decision-support and development efforts in physician systems to identify areas of importance in the design of systems for medication management and drug decision support at the point of care.

The Problems

A variety of issues contribute to the rising cost of healthcare as well as to difficulties with clinical information management. We present several issues here.

Costs. The national annual cost of drug-related morbidity and mortality is estimated to be as high as $76.6 billion. About $47 billion of that is attributed just to hospital admissions associated with drug therapy or the absence of appropriate drug therapy. By comparison, the cost of diabetes care has been estimated at $45.2 billion.[2]

Legal Claims. Drug injuries frequently result in malpractice claims, and in a large study of adjudicated claims, drug injuries accounted for the highest total expenditure of any type of procedure-related injury.[3]

Marketing by Drug Companies. Drug costs in health maintenance organizations (HMOs) increased 25 percent in recent years.[4] A contributing factor to this steep rise is the prescribing of more expensive and sometimes less effective medications that are being successfully marketed to physicians.[5][6][7]

Nonadherence to Clinical Guidelines. Physicians and prescribers, for reasons that go beyond the scope of this discussion, seldom follow even well-established clinical guidelines for care and prescribing.[8][9]

The Solution

Many concerned with both the economic and the medical consequences of this problem have called for physicians to use direct, computerized order-entry systems for prescribing. In 1995 the American Society of Health-System Pharmacists established a policy of supporting, "as the preferred method of prescribing, direct electronic entry of medication orders by the prescriber." The National Coordinating Council for Medication Error Reporting and Prevention urged the use of direct, computerized order entry to address the most common cause of prescription errors.[10] An editorial in the *Journal of the American Medical Association* states, "Computer interventions with drug-associated errors and other errors in medicine should continue to be developed, implemented and evaluated."[11] A more recent editorial states that "computerized prescribing in the practice of medicine is a change that is overdue."[12] These recommendations are made on the assumption that a decision-support system will inform physicians of an adverse event prior to its occurrence and will advise on proper drug therapy at the point of care.

Studies have shown the value of electronic ordering systems in decreasing the number of adverse drug events,[13][14] dropping infection rates,[15] improving dosing,[16] increasing generic prescribing and formulary compliance,[17] and decreasing the cost of care.[18][19] Brigham and Women's Hospital reports savings of up to $10 million annually by using computerized order entry.[20] In one study 23 percent of all the adverse events were judged to have been preventable if electronic ordering systems had been in place.[21] In a follow-up study, the number of serious medication errors was reduced by 55 percent when physicians used a computer order-entry system.[22] Thus, the use of medication order-entry systems at the point of care, with decision support to influence drug-therapy cost and quality, is clearly indicated.[23] A number of issues need to be addressed in the evaluation, development, implementation, and ongoing support of electronic ordering systems.

Issues

In considering CDS for medication management several issues need to be addressed: the clinical setting and physician workflow, commercial DUR/DUE alerting programs, customer alerts, formulary, and knowledge representation. We discuss each of these in turn.

Inpatient Versus Outpatient Prescribing. The problem with extrapolating the results of many of these studies to most nonhospital-based practices is twofold. First, most were designed and carried out in a hospital setting, and, second, the decision-support logic was customized by the reporting institutions. It is important to question whether these impressive results will be realized when plug-and-play commercial products are used in the outpatient setting, where most prescribing takes place. Physician workflow and use of electronic prescribing in the office environment are vastly different than they are in hospitals and hospital-based clinics. Few outpatient organizations have the expertise to develop drug-utilization review and/or evaluation (DUR/DUE) and therefore may not reproduce the positive results seen in nonambulatory studies. Therefore, despite the recognized benefits of this technology, relatively few applications are in use in physician offices to facilitate prescription writing.[24]

Physician Workflow. Physician workflow and computer use are complex and variable. The largest issue with the automation of prescription writing is simply speed. Although the benefits are compelling, getting prescribers (mostly physicians) to use electronic methods of ordering is a challenge because of time pressures. A prescriber can scribble a drug name and directions on a readily available prescription pad much more quickly than finding a computer, logging on, filling in all the needed fields, and electronically signing the order. It is unlikely that stand-alone electronic prescription writers that add no value to the prescribing practice will be successful. However, a system that within the workflow of the physician points out potential problems, tracks previous medications, and automates renewals more than compensates for the extra time involved in making an electronic order entry.

Commercial Alerting Programs. Various commercial vendors of tools for clinical decision support have produced databases of drugs and knowledge bases to embed in ordering systems. Typically they offer drug-drug, drug-allergy, drug-condition, drug-pregnancy, drug-pediatric, duration-of-therapy and therapeutic-duplication alerts. Mounting evidence indicates that these systems may not be working with the effectiveness of the customized systems at the point of care.

These commercially available DUR/DUE alerting systems may not produce information that is clinically relevant at the point of care. The reasons include the inability of the system to individualize the patient and to identify those elements of the patient's medication and medical history that affect prescription ordering. Many medications on the market typically have a binary action. If a patient is on one drug or has one disease and an interacting drug is prescribed, an alert is fired. For example, such systems will inform only of interactions between Drug A and Drug B, not of the effects of Drugs A, C, D, and E on Drug B. Disease conditions affecting liver, renal, and other organs are rarely taken into account in determining interacting drugs and therapies. In many cases interactions are dose-dependent—they occur only when a certain dose is reached.

False alarms and the frequent appearance of unnecessary verbiage, or "clinical noise," can lead to the prescriber's ignoring alerts that do have clinical significance. They can also cause user frustration with the applications. For instance, the use of outpatient prescription writers utilizing commercially available DUR/DUE alerts in Veterans Administration institutions inhibited use of the system.[25]

Congress passed the Omnibus Budget Reconciliation Act in 1990, requiring states to provide claims-based drug-utilization review at the point of dispensing for approximately thirty-four million Medicaid enrollees. It was believed that this action could promote safety and reduce costs, and these results have been shown in some of the reports in the literature.[26] These commercially available DUR/DUE systems have been implemented in pharmacy benefit-management systems for checking claims and in retail pharmacy systems for checking prescriptions at the time of dispensing.[27] There is considerable debate in the pharmacy and physician community about whether this type of DUR/DUE checking has any value.[28][29] No valid scientific data support the claimed benefits of these commercially available, computer-based DUR/DUE alerts.[30] These same alerting systems are being widely implemented in prescription-writing products without regard for either therapeutic benefits or physician acceptance.

If an alert is truly useful and patient-specific, the desired result would be to take action on the recommendation stated. In the usual case of writing a prescription and receiving a drug-drug, drug-allergy, drug-condition, drug-pregnancy, drug-pediatric, duration-of-therapy or therapeutic-duplication alert, a change in the medication prescribed would result. Therefore, measuring the incidence of changed orders at the time of alert would be an indication of the usefulness the alert. If the rate of acceptance of the suggested or implied change in therapy is low, it may be that the clinical noise is too high and is having a negative impact on usability.

Studies have been made of DUR/DUE alerts presented to pharmacists and the action taken. In two studies, alerts appeared in 9.1 to 19 percent of prescriptions processed at the point of dispensing in state Medicaid populations.[31][32] Of these prescriptions, 20.9 percent and 4 percent, respectively, were not dispensed. In the larger study prescriptions were dispensed 17.7 percent of the time after the pharmacist contacted the prescriber, in 20.6 percent of cases after the pharmacist talked with the patient, and 37.2 percent of the time after a review of internal resources.

Extrapolating these data to anticipate behavior at the point of care raises some important usability issues. The expected result of a change in therapy (where a physician prescriber instead of a pharmacist initiates a cancellation of the order) would be expected to occur the same percentage of the time an alert is presented (4 and 20.9 percent). Taking the worst case, from a usability standpoint, if a prescriber sees an alert in 19 percent of the orders and takes action only 4 percent of the time, the user will perceive that the system has a high level of clinical noise and therefore will not consider the system useful. Even the best case yields an alert 9.1 percent of the time and a change in therapy 20 percent of the time.

The "perfect" clinical alerting system could be described as one in which every alert was clinically appropriate and accurate enough to trigger a change in the ordered medication. If it is assumed that using current systems, a change in therapy based on alerts occurs only 4 to 20 percent of the time, the alert clearly has less than perfect impact. It could be that the clinical inferences contained in the alert have less meaning to the pharmacist than they would to the physician at the point of care, who knows the specifics of the patient's condition. It is possible that the incidence of therapy change after presentation of DUR/DUE alerts would be higher at the point of care than at the point of dispensing. If alerts are clinically significant and reflective of the patient's medical condition, an increase in acceptance and a subsequent change in therapy could be anticipated. The time and frustration involved when the pharmacist has to call the physician after getting an alert are largely eliminated when the alert is presented initially to the prescriber. If the alerts presented by any system are not clinically relevant, change in therapy rates will be low and therefore will contribute to clinical noise. More studies need to be done prior to the widespread acceptance and use of many of the current plug-and-play decision-support systems.

Custom Alerts. Ultimately organizations will need to implement care guidelines and rules in an automated system that has local acceptance and is applicable to their own patient population. Unfortunately, it is not easy to accomplish this goal by implementing currently available, off-the-shelf commercial products. For example, it is well accepted that a rising potassium in combination with the heart drug digoxin should result in action. Some physicians, however, like to run potassium "a little high" with patients. An alert will have to qualify and quantify what "a little high" means if the system is to meet with the approval of a subset of physicians. Producing care alerts that are widely accepted and relevant is an arduous and complex process. An explanation of one process methodology has been previously published.[33] Although a number of vendors provide the tools by which to customize alerts, few organizations and practices to date have taken the initiative to fully utilize these logic tools. It is far easier, of course, to use off-the-shelf solutions provided by decision-support vendors and hope for effective therapeutic results. As more benefit studies emerge, the value will become more apparent, and more organizations will make the investment of time and personnel needed to create useful and medically correct decision-support rules and alerts. An organization proceeding without an understanding of the need to implement and support custom medication rules and alerts and without providing them would be shortsighted.

Formularies and Plan Design. There are as many formularies and drug-benefit designs as there are organizations managing them. Knowing what drugs are covered and the circumstances under which they are covered and knowing how to represent those concepts on the screen is a design and support issue. Because benefit managers often feel that plan design is essential to their competitive advantage, it is sometimes difficult to find out all the specifics of a plan in order to describe them properly. There is currently no central source of complete information on all the following concepts. Therefore the only practical solution is to go directly to the plans represented in a population, obtain the information, and set up mechanisms for updating the decision-support system.

Formulary Types. There are open, closed, and other types of formularies. In open formularies technically no items are not covered; however, many items have a preferred status. In closed formularies a specified set of drugs is covered and not covered. There are also a variety of open formularies with closed categories of medications (such as oral contraceptives or other types of medications).

Preferred Status. A class of drugs may contain a preferred drug for reimbursement and targeting therapeutic-switching campaigns. Within a therapeutic class one or two drugs may be the only ones covered by the benefit plan.

Drugs Not Preferred. With or without a preferred drug in a class there may be drugs that are *not* preferred. With an open formulary the plan may pay for the drug but display messages to the pharmacist at the time of dispensing and ask for a call to the physician when refills are due in order to switch from the not-preferred medication to the preferred drug.

Second-Line Agents. These medications will be paid for only if one or more other agents, typically in the same therapeutic class, have been tried and treatment has failed. There may be time requirements for the previous course of treatment.

Therapeutic Alternatives. There may be a drug in the same class or another class that is preferred over the target medication.

Prior Authorization. The plan may pay for the drug only under very specific circumstances, which may depend on a patient's concurrent or previous disease states.

Variable Copay. There are now multiple copayments based on whether the medication is preferred, not preferred, generic, a single-source brand (only one supplier), or cobranded (brand drug available from more than one manufacturer).

Knowledge Representation and Nomenclature. The following representational concepts are a challenge to implement and evaluate in an automated order-entry system. Each drug database, obtained either directly from the Food and Drug Administration (FDA) or indirectly from one of the commercial vendors, needs careful design in order to limit the selection possibilities so that the database is easy to use but does not unreasonably restrict the medications the prescriber can order.

Generic Drug. Maximizing generic prescribing can have a huge impact on decreasing costs. A desirable feature in a system is the express order on the prescription to dispense the drug with a generic product. Knowing what drugs are available generically in a database is not straightforward. The FDA tags each drug it regulates with a code known as the Orange Book Code because it is published in an orange book. Any drug with an "A" in its code has been shown to be generically equivalent. There may be a significant time lag from the "A" rating of a drug to its actual use because of manufacturing and distribution time. Some benefit plans, however, only recognize the list published by the Health Care Financing Administration (HCFA) and assign a maximum allowable cost (MAC). Even though a drug is "A"-rated, there is a time lag before it is on the HCFA MAC list. As if these considerations did not make database design difficult enough, some states publish a list of drugs they deem generically equivalent. So, if a system used only the Orange Book Code to interpret generic equivalency, the drug might not be available in the pharmacy, might not be paid for by the plan, or might not even be legal in certain states.

Brand Drug. Typically a brand drug is one that has been marketed by the innovator with a name that is easier to say and write than the chemical or generic name. Some manufacturers may allow other manufacturers to market the identical product under yet another brand name. One of these cobranded products may even be a preferred or not preferred product by a specific plan, further complicating the issue for the prescriber.

National Drug Codes. The National Drug Code (NDC) is the only nonproprietary numbering sequence published by the FDA. It is completely inadequate for decision-support design, primarily because the codes are different for identical drugs from different manufacturers and in different package sizes. For a more detailed description of NDC and other concepts the reader is referred to the "Unauthorized Lexicon Guide" available at www.multum.com.

The Health Level Seven Committee is working to establish a more robust standard drug vocabulary for the industry. Any agreement with a database vendor should include a commitment to map to the emerging standard so that the organization does not get locked into one database vendor.

Electronic Transfer, Faxing, and Printing of Prescriptions. Most pharmacy vendors and chains have not enabled their system to accept prescriptions via one of the competing standards for electronic prescriptions (Script from the National Council for Prescription Drug Programs and MedPre from the American Society for Automation in Pharmacy). With the majority of states allowing faxed prescriptions it would seem logical for most pharmacies to have fax machines, but even in large metropolitan areas only about 40 percent of pharmacies do.[34] Presumably, retail pharmacies make a fair amount of profit from nonmedication sales while people wait for prescriptions, and therefore they have little incentive to speed up the process.

Some states have strict requirements for the color, font size, specific language, and location of verbiage on printed prescriptions. It is therefore necessary for designers to take into account individual state requirements in order for their products to be widely acceptable.

Conclusion

Adverse drug events (ADEs) and benefit-plan compliance are major contributors to poor therapeutic outcomes and to the soaring cost of pharmaceutical care. There has been a proliferation of prescription ordering systems that contain commercially available DUR/DUE. Unfortunately, use of most of these systems has not made a significant impact on the rate of ADEs or on cost in part because of the current practice of placing alerts at the point of dispensing rather than presenting them to the prescriber and in part because the alert is often inappropriate for the specific clinical situation for which a medication is ordered.

Any solution utilizing electronic decision support must move the alerting system from the point of dispensing to the point of prescribing, be applicable to the widest spectrum of clinical situations, and enable the prescriber to take the specific requirements of the patient into account.

References

1. Lazarou, J., Pomeranz, B. H., and Corey, P. N. "Incidence of Adverse Drug Reactions in Hospitalized Patients." *Journal of the American Medical Association,* 1998, *279,* 1200–1205.
2. Johnson, J. A., and Bootman, J. L. "Drug-Related Morbidity and Mortality: A Cost-of-Illness Model." *Archives of Internal Medicine,* 1995, *155,* 1949–1956.
3. National Association of Insurance Commissioners. *Medical Malpractice Claims (Closed), 1975–1978.* Kansas City: NAIC, 1979.
4. Frazier, G. "Strategies to Tackle Recent Surge in Pharmacy Costs." *Drug Benefit Trends,* 1997, *9* (11), 31–49.
5. Soumerai, S. B. "Principles and Uses of Academic Detailing to Improve the Management of Psychiatric Disorders." *International Journal of Psychiatry in Medicine,* 1998, *28* (1), 81–96.
6. Brufsky, J. W., Ross-Degnan, D., Calabrese, D., Gao, X., and Soumerai, S. B. "Shifting Physician Prescribing to a Preferred Histamine-2-Receptor Antagonist: Effects of a Multifactorial Intervention in a Mixed-Model Health Maintenance Organization." *Medical Care,* 1998, *36* (3), 321–332.
7. "Is Good Marketing Bad Medicine?" *Business Week,* Apr. 13, 1998, pp. 62–63.
8. Lantner, R. R., and Ros, S. P. "Emergency Management of Asthma in Children: Impact of NIH Guidelines." *Annals of Allergy Asthma and Immunology,* 1995, *74,* 188–191.
9. Berlowitz, D. R., and others, "Inadequate Management of Blood Pressure in a Hypertensive Population." *New England Journal of Medicine,* 1998, *339,* 27.
10. "Recommendations to Reduce Rx Errors." *American Druggist,* 1996, *213,* 18.
11. Kahn, K. L. "Above All 'Do No Harm': How Shall We Avoid Errors in Medicine?" *Journal of the American Medical Association,* 1995, *274,* 75–76.
12. Schiff, G. D., and Rucker, T. D. "Computerized Prescribing: Building the Electronic Infrastructure for Better Medication Usage." *Journal of the American Medical Association,* 1998, *279,* 1024–1029.
13. Evans, R. S., and others. "Using a Hospital Information System to Assess the Effects of Adverse Drug Events." *Proceedings of the Annual Symposium on Computer Applications in Medical Care,* 1993, *17,* 161–165.
14. Classen, D. C., Pestotnik, S. L., Evans, R. S., and Burke, J. P. "Computerized Surveillance of Adverse Drug Events in Hospital Patients." *Journal of the American Medical Association,* 1991, *266,* 2847–2878.

15. Evans, R. S., and others. "Computer Surveillance of Hospital-Acquired Infections and Antibiotic Use." *Journal of the American Medical Association,* 1986, *256* (8), 1007–1011.

16. Lenert, L., Sheiner, L., and Blaschke, T. F. "Improving Drug Dosing in Hospitalized Patients: Automated Modeling of Pharmacokinetics for Drug Dosing Regimens." *Proceedings of the 12th Annual Symposium on Computer Applications in Medical Care,* 1988, 238–312.

17. Rivkin, S. "Opportunities and Challenges of Electronic Physician Prescribing Technology." *Medical Interface,* 1997, *10,* 77–80, 83.

18. Tierney, W. M., Miller, M. E., Overhage, J. M., and McDonald, C. J. "Physician Inpatient Order Writing on Microcomputer Workstations: Effects on Resource Utilization." *Journal of the American Medical Association,* 1993, *269,* 379–383.

19. Pestotnik, S. L., Classen, D. C., Evans, S. R., and Burke, J. P. "Implementing Antibiotic Practice Guidelines Through Computer-Assisted Decision Support: Clinical and Financial Outcomes." *Annals of Internal Medicine,* 1996, *124,* 884–889.

20. Glaser, J., and Kuperman, G. J. "Impact of Information Events on Medical Care." *Proceedings of the Healthcare Information Management Systems Society Conference,* 1996, *2,* 2–9.

21. Bates, D. W., O'Neil, A. C., Boyle, D., Teich, J., Chertow, G. M., Komaroff, A. L., and Brennan, T. A. "Potential Identifiability and Preventability of Adverse Events Using Information Systems." *Journal of the American Medical Informatics Association,* 1994, *1,* 404–411.

22. Bates, W. B., Leape, L. L., Cullen, D. J., Laird, N., Peterson, L. A., and Teich, J. M. "Effect of Computerized Physician Order Entry and a Team Intervention on Prevention of Serious Medication Errors." *Journal of the American Medical Association,* 1998, *280,* 1311–1316.

23. Garibaldi, R. A. "Computers and the Quality of Care: A Clinician's Perspective." *New England Journal of Medicine,* 1998, *338,* 259–260.

24. Reich, P. R. "Formulary Wars." *Managed Care Interface,* 1998, *11,* 14.

25. Powell, V. "Computerized Physician Outpatient Prescription Order Entry: Department of Defense's Version." *Hospital Pharmacy,* 1997, *32,* 65–74.

26. U.S. General Accounting Office. *Prescription Drugs and Medicaid Automated Review Systems Can Help Promote Safety, Save Money.* GAO/AIMD-96-72. Gaithersburg, Md.: U.S. General Accounting Office, 1996.

27. Schulman, K. A. "The Effect of Pharmaceutical Benefit Managers: Is It Being Evaluated?" *Annals of Internal Medicine,* 1996, *124,* 906–913.

28. McGuffey, E. C. "Computerized DUR Alerts: Boon or Bane to Pharmaceutical Care." *Journal of the American Pharmacy Associates,* 1998, *38,* 122–124.

29. Soumerai, S. B., McLaughlin, T. J., and Avorn, J. "Improving Drug Prescribing in Primary Care: A Critical Analysis of the Experimental Literature." *Milbank Quarterly,* 1989, *67* (2), 268–317.

30. Soumerai, S. B., and Lipton, H. L. Computer-Based Drug-Utilization Review—Risk, Benefit or Boondoggle. *New England Journal of Medicine,* 1996, *332,* 1641–1645.

31. Armstrong, E. P., and Denmark, C. R. "How Pharmacists Respond to Online, Real Time DUR Alerts." *Journal of the American Pharmacy Associates,* 1998, *38,* 149–154.

32. McPeak, M. E. "State-by-State Look at Medicaid Retail Pharmacy Delivery: Trial and Triumphs." *Journal of Managed Care Pharmaceuticals,* 1998, *4,* 546–554.

33. Guzman, S., Jamieson, P. W., Poikonen, J., and Smith, J. "The Development of Clinical Alerts for Managing Care." *Proceedings of the Healthcare Information Management Systems Society Conference,* 1997, *1,* 393–404.

34. Sardinha, C. "Electronic Prescribing: The Next Revolution in Pharmacy?" *Journal of Managed Care Pharmaceuticals,* 1998, *4,* 35–39.

About the Authors

John Poikonen, R.Ph., is a system designer and clinical content specialist at Synetic Healthcare Communication, Inc., Cambridge, Massachusetts, and a Doctor of Pharmacy Candidate at Nova Southeastern University.

John M. Leventhal, M.D., is the physician executive of Synetic Healthcare Communication, Inc. He has over twenty-five years of experience in the clinical practice of surgery, obstetrics, and gynecology and as a faculty member at the Harvard Medical School.

Disease Management and Clinical Decision Support

*Rufus S. Howe, F.N.P.; Michael B. Terpening;
Sandeep Wadhwa, M.D., M.B.A.*

The term *disease management* is so broad that it covers essentially all aspects of clinical medicine. Indeed, the disparate range of care activities that are touted under its banner would appear to demonstrate the term's vacuity. Despite the unfortunate moniker, however, the underlying concepts of disease management may ultimately transform how healthcare is organized and delivered. Disease management is probably best understood if viewed as the offspring of the total quality management (TQM) and the cost-control movements of the 1980s.[1][2] Its central tenets are a disease-specific focus, quality improvement, and cost efficiency. To date, most efforts have succeeded only in being disease-specific. This article discusses the central role that clinical decision support (CDS) plays in creating and demonstrating the value of disease management.

Historical Overview

The disease-specific focus of these efforts arises from the insights that are gained from analyzing the natural history of disease processes. In general, healthcare systems are superbly poised to address acute illnesses. However, the bulk of illnesses are chronic and are characterized by a slow, debilitating course marked with episodes of acute decompensation.[3] Intervening after the event is incredibly expensive. When processes are targeted earlier, health is maintained and costly complications are avoided. By the same token, well-intentioned early interventions for patients with low risk of developing decompensation also result in resource expenditures without proof of a beneficial impact. Many prenatal programs targeted at healthy mothers exemplify this problem.[4] These programs are probably of greater benefit for their marketing, actuarial, or regulatory value than for their affect on health.[5]

The salient observation is that a small portion of the population consumes a disproportionately large share of health care resources.[6] The task of CDS is not only to provide insights into disease processes in order to identify opportunities to intercede earlier but also to identify the individuals who are most likely to develop complications. A key benefit therefore of using decision-support tools in disease management is their ability to target focused interventions according to the severity of the patient's condition.

The second component of disease management is its incorporation of quality-improvement efforts. A host of quality-management gurus—Walter Shewart, W. Edwards Deming, Joseph M. Juran, and Philip B. Crosby—articulated a series of quality principles that changed industrial operations in the 1970s and 1980s.[7] The 1980s and 1990s then saw the application of these principles in the service sector. Key features of the quality movement are the primacy of customer satisfaction, staff empowerment, process measurement and variation control, and commitment to minimize rework. A clear message from the movement is that investments in quality pay off in either lower costs or higher revenues. Healthcare industry practitioners who initially applied the principles of TQM introduced quality circles and multidisciplinary teams. The elements of TQM that disease management emphasizes are measurement, variation control, and attention to patient needs. Perhaps the clearest example has been the proliferation of guidelines and clinical pathways. Concern for process variation is based on the dramatic deviation in clinical practice. Guidelines were developed to minimize care variation by establishing codified approaches that could then be embedded in decision-support systems used by clinicians to help ensure consistent care delivery across large patient panels with disease-specific conditions. Developers are now further refining the tools of CDS to seamlessly integrate the guidelines and pathways into the clinician's workflow. Disease-management efforts have resulted in disease mapping, evidence-based protocols, and best-practice approaches. However, efforts have yet to focus as critically on process measurement and outcomes management. Only by understanding the impact of an interventions will one be able to judge its value. Determining the appropriate outcomes and developing the systems that track outcomes are central tasks of CDS.

The third component of disease-management programs is the focus on reducing or controlling costs. This goal has been somewhat elusive to date. Program costs are high, and such initiatives cannot be directly linked to generating revenue or reducing costs quickly enough to satisfy the six- to twelve-month expectations of financial decision makers. Program costs are also particularly prone to both labor and technology overruns. Reimbursement is problematic too, as it is generally focused only on problem solving and acute episodes. When such services are reimbursed, as is case-management education, monitoring, and preventive maintenance, payment is low. Furthermore, inferior program design, low retention, poor physician acceptance, and inadequate tracking of patients and outcomes further degrade the value proposition.

The various stakeholders in the disease-management process include patients, providers, employers and purchasers, pharmaceutical and device suppliers, and institutional providers such as integrated delivery networks.

Each participant, though, operates with different incentives that have yet to be successfully aligned.[8] For example, disease-management initiatives seek to reduce excessive and unnecessary doctor visits and hospitalizations; however, discounted fee for service and the prospective-payment system motivate providers to increase visits or hospitalizations. The misaligned incentives and the difficulty of putting programs into operation have forced a host of firms to leave the disease-management industry. These are formidable barriers, and it may require time to overcome them before payers change reimbursement patterns. Unfortunately though, until further evidence proves the interventions' effectiveness, these barriers will likely remain. In spite of the challenges, CDS promises to play a critical role in managing the costs, operational design, and implementation of these programs.

Standards and Methods

CDS is nothing more than providing the appropriate information to the right audience at the most opportune time. Decision-support systems are based on warehousing data from multiple sources and delivering data that highlight pivotal factors. Evidence suggests that significant health improvements can occur when patients suffering from chronic diseases are provided with personalized reminders and targeted information about their condition and have access to advice from caregivers.[9]

In a healthcare environment, a patient may move from physician to physician, in and out of inpatient and outpatient settings, and from health plan to health plan, and it is extremely complicated to keep clinical data flowing among these constituencies. Contributing to the challenge of data sharing is the dearth of standards that are adhered to by the key players—providers, hospitals, and health plans—for identifying members and passing clinical data. The lack of a universal standard has created competing solutions ranging from computerized patient-record sets to proprietary interfaces built by private healthcare companies to bridge the gaps.

Rather than wait for global answers, forward-thinking organizations are building partnerships and working with emerging technical standards. These partnerships provide the mutual benefits of patient improvement, cost-effective use of healthcare resources, and data reporting that can meet the requirements of the Joint Commission on Accreditation of Healthcare Organizations and the National Committee for Quality Assurance.

Partnerships of plans, providers, outsourcing groups, and community resources have become possible because the technology now offers simplified interfaces, encapsulation of legacy data, and ubiquitous access from public and private intranets and extranets as well as the Internet. These data partnerships leverage existing claims, billing, and patient and provider demographic-data feeds that pass between the constituent caregivers and payers.

Foundations of Clinical Decision Support. Effective CDS for disease management hinges on these foundations:

- Consistent identification of data elements for inputs
- Standards for data formats and system protocols
- Data-warehousing infrastructure (databases, network connectivity, access methods)
- Identification of user profiles and data proximity needs
- Practice-guideline and clinical-decision logic to feed the alerts, triggers, and trending reports
- Appropriate timing of data delivery

Identification of Data Elements and Supporting Standards. A master patient index (MPI) is critical to the success of any longitudinal trending. It is essential that all the data contributors track people as they travel in and out of plan coverage.[10]

The organization must undertake an analysis of available data. The most effective clinical-decision warehouse would include the following elements:

Information from health-risk assessments. A number of vehicles are available based on variations of the standard SF12 questions or National Health Information Survey forms.

Health-plan claims data from facilities and physician offices. These records are rich with ICD-9, CPT-4, and disease-related-group codes and are of critical value in long-term trending—American National Standards Institute standards, Accredited Standards Committee (ASC) X12, Health Level Seven.

Prescription data from pharmacy claims passed in standard formats: ASC X12, National Council of Prescription Drug Programs telecom standard v3.2, American Society for Automation in Pharmacy MedPre prescription Electronic Data Interchange standard.

Clinical-criteria review data used in admission, procedure, and specialist-referral authorizations. These data are more timely than claims data and offer inputs for the alerts and triggers.

Telemetry-transmitted home medical devices with remote modem connectivity to base units. More and more of these devices are becoming available for home monitoring of chronic conditions.

Records from acute-episode triage-nurse lines. The advent of advice-nurse lines and demand-management algorithm-based triage has created a new body of data on patients' acute episodes. These data can signal potential troubles from patient-reported high-risk symptoms. The most clinically rigorous systems gather details on patient-reported conditions along with corresponding indicators about diagnoses that cannot be ruled out in triage sessions. A fairly large percentage (30 to 40) of the triage calls may result in patient self-care instructions that would ordinarily be lost to the claims system.

Users and Access. Access to the data store is provided to the following key participants in the disease-management process:

Providers who are involved directly in treating the individual patient must be provided access to details from all the sources.

Case managers access details to follow individuals' progress and confirm clinical intensity for procedure and admission certifications.

Triage and disease-management nurses have access to the system for the purpose of adjusting patient-education materials or increasing the frequency of monitoring.

Patients can be allowed a top-line view of their treatment history with links to the textual medical information and self-care instructions.

Warehousing. A comprehensive data store receives contributions from all the key players and provides health-condition, history, and progress data for trending and raising predefined alerts. The warehouse does not need to exist at a single location. Multiple data sources can be polled from a web-based application to combine data elements into a single display, especially for patient-information text that can be effectively linked from external sources. Each data source should be examined to determine whether the data are bundled to a data-mart server indexed by a Master Patient Index or whether the patient data can be queried directly from the web application.

Connectivity is not the main concern for data sharing in this manner. A web application can control the piping of data for single patients indexed by the MPI fairly quickly. The new concerns are ensuring that data are secure and are delivered with the appropriate level of detail.

Security. A fire-walled intranet in which all users have a secure physical connection is the most secure delivery method for this disease-management clinical decision support system (CDSS). Such a model supports a single location and perhaps a single managing entity, but a partnership of companies is more likely to decentralize the warehouse with virtual private networks that provide encrypted channels across common Internet conduits. Improvements in secure web channels provide strong protection for most patient records. Enforced password protection and a relatively short time-out cycle to close are essential to this effort.

Proposed Network. Figure 1 is a diagram of a possible network for CDS; it incorporates the standards and methods discussed here.

Critical Functionality

An effective CDS must handle the transfer of clinical data to all the participants, evaluate that data against best clinical practices, and raise predefined alerts and trigger follow-up events.

A full body of clinical-guideline and best-practice data are available in citations and in care-management software systems for the most costly disease states such as asthma, diabetes, hypertension, and congestive heart disease. In

Figure 1. Proposed Network for Clinical Decision Support

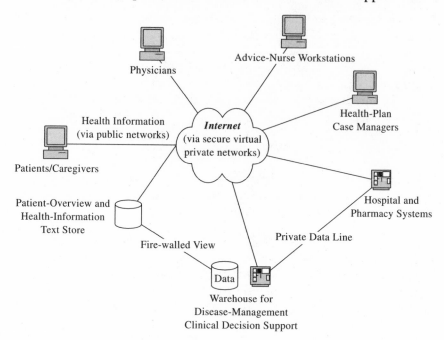

addition to these sources, a wealth of information is recorded during clinical-care criteria-review sessions authorizing procedures by the utilization and case-management or review departments.

Physicians may be the first to know about medications, inpatient admissions, and laboratory findings, but often they are not aware of patient-education efforts, nurse triage information, or health-risk-appraisal outcomes. Physicians in traditional managed-care arrangements are often not aware of all the health-plan authorization criteria until they are contacted for clarification. Providing the physician with these data will help with disease monitoring.

Case managers can also benefit from the progress notes on patient education and the prevention reminders that an automated CDS can provide. Results of continued-stay utilization-management reviews for inpatient activity can be made available long before actual claims data arrive.

After the cogent data elements are identified in the warehouse, they are mapped against clinical-guideline logic so that sets of Boolean logic statements can be applied against the data to create a knowledge base. The logic statements need not be much more complex than combinations of data elements and ranges linked to proposed actions. The power of the CDS originates from the rigor of the clinical content and not from any complex computations.

Some trigger indicators from the clinical guidelines will not be defined by the inputs received. The partnering organizations must determine whether it is important to institute incremental data gathering for those elements.

Decision-triggering logic applies data from as many of the data sources as possible against a set of treatment-plan elements and the knowledge base to determine severity. Severity scores specific to each disease set determine the appropriate core content for clinical best practices in the treatment of the disease as well as patient- and caregiver-education materials.

The CDS mines the data warehoused as raw materials to calculate the severity level of the patient's chronic condition and to trigger recommendations. These are the specific functions of the system:

- Calculates severity-level trends
- Indicates appropriate patient-education materials or home devices
- Generates reminders for regular provider visits, medication reviews, and laboratory testing
- Compares pharmacy data against standard prescription recommendations from citations and local standards as well as highlights any possible adverse drug interactions
- Recommends appropriate alternate locations for care as needs change
- Assesses trends in patients' attitude and mental health
- Queues e-mail, snail mail, or fax reminders to the physician, case manager, or patient
- Generates outbound telephonic task actions for advice nurses in a comprehensive disease-management environment (advice nurses provide the personal contact that reinforces the patient-based recommendations)

Impact of Decision-Support Tools in Disease Management

From the quality-management point of view, the systems that support disease management represent a significant step forward in measuring and improving longitudinal care. An understanding of how a person carries out diabetes care from month to month, year to year, is not easily obtainable today.

One way of evaluating the impact on disease management is to consider some major domains of care: clinical parameters, knowledge, behavior, utilization, and satisfaction.

Clinical data points can be separated into two distinct types, subjective and objective. Subjective data include symptoms; measured data include blood pressure, for example. Changes in clinical data are obvious evidence of impact. The problems many disease-management services face are the reliability of observational data—especially data provided over the telephone—and access to measured data. Another challenge is in the area of sampling. Because clinical measurement is a "snapshot" and may not reflect the true severity of the condition, trending these data becomes a paramount consideration, and it is expensive. We will see below how remote monitoring can play an important role.

Both physician and patient knowledge is a factor in disease management.[11] Profiling both groups for knowledge is an interesting exercise. Physicians may not be aware of the latest medications, diagnostic tests, or resources. Patients are not likely to have adequate self-management knowledge.[12] Measuring knowledge is a challenge with both groups, but it is helpful in tracking the effectiveness of the educational aspect of the program.

Changes in behaviors that lead to health-promoting or health-demoting results are important to track. Behaviors include smoking, avoidance of asthma aggravators, alcohol consumption, and exercise. The pitfall of this domain is its self-reported nature. Many physicians are skeptical and discount this form of data.

Changes in utilization data are crucial for the renewal of a disease-management program from an economic standpoint. The reliability and validity of claims data are being seriously questioned across the board, however. Coding problems, timeliness of claims, and specificity in assigning the claim (such as it is) to the condition in question are some of the limitations associated with claims-based studies.

Satisfaction data are as good as the satisfaction tool. Satisfaction is a moving target and can be heavily influenced by the interviewer, the subject's mood, and the quality of the question itself. Nevertheless, satisfaction continues to be a valuable measure of program quality.

On a purely operational level, disease management promises to have an impact in at least three areas—problem identification, information sharing, and logistical support. Designed well, applications that meet the functional characteristics mentioned in the previous section should satisfy these requirements. Designed poorly, the application will be nothing more than a glorified "smart form." Unfortunately, current disease-management applications more closely resemble the latter.

Problem identification. From the payer's perspective, one of the most valuable aspects of a disease-management program is its ability to troll the targeted population for emerging or actual problematic patients. The clinical and economic impact of early identification of potential or real problems is immense. Accomplishing this task is daunting, and it requires both a proactive and reactive component.

Proactive problem identification involves designing an alert and reminder system for persons who are in an at-risk or high-risk state. From a clinical point of view, we know the characteristics of members who demand regular attention. Examples include review of downloadable home monitoring devices and regularly scheduled outbound calls.

Reactive problem identification sounds contradictory, but it is not. The hallmark of successful patient education is problem-solving abilities. If patients are able to identify warning signs of impending problems (elevated blood-glucose levels for diabetics, weight gain for persons with congestive heart failure), then they can act on what they know. Again, the systems that monitor this activity are an integral part of helping people validate the urgency of the situation.

Information sharing. The possibility of changing behavior on the basis of newly learned or relearned information has always been in doubt. The old adage "knowledge doesn't necessarily lead to behavior" holds true even in the face of the most sophisticated application. The key point is to design a system that supports multiple methods of information giving. More impact can be predicted with a system that includes personal telephone conversations, general and customized written information, and all manner of web-based media.

Logistical support. Helping persons with a chronic illness wade through the unending cycle of keeping medical appointments, obtaining durable medical equipment, dealing with reimbursement structures, and other social elements is invaluable. The case-management literature is filled with examples of cost avoidance when care for people with chronic illnesses is coordinated.[13][14]

Future Trends

While the impact of CDS on disease management today may occur in the ways described above, in the future other ways will be seen as well. Cooperative ROI, person-based systems, physician-driven or patient monitor design, data integration, increased data from remote sites, and multiple ports of entry all represent new ways in which CDS may impact disease management.

Cooperative Return on Investment. Certainly, all parties involved with a disease-management program will be motivated to prove value. More and more clients are asking for consultative services that help them think through the logic of the intervention and feel comfortable that it will drive costs down, improve their health status, and be a caring, person-based program.

Future efforts in this area will include a bevy of data-sharing options. Exhibit 1 is a form for supplying data for a prospective diabetes disease-management program. Obviously, this form will require that the client have access to reliable claims data; these data will not only identify patients but will stratify them into risk categories. If the client does not have reliable claims data, the client and the disease manager must make assumptions that have to be rechecked at a later date.

On a related note, predictive models that are able to accurately list next year's high-cost patients will proliferate in the coming years. Today's models are able to accurately identify approximately 35 percent of the next year's high-risk patients. Unfortunately, some psychics have a higher accuracy rate, so we clearly have a way to go.

Person-Based Systems. The market will no longer tolerate disease-specific programs. Newer programs will seamlessly integrate multiple comorbid conditions filtering out redundancy of data points to reach their logical conclusion in a plan of care.

Exhibit 1. Form for Supplying Data for a Prospective Diabetes Disease-Management Program

Number of members in plan: _____

Estimated percent of population with diabetes: _____

Estimated percent of above population to enroll: _____

Percent of members with each classification (should be equal to 100):

Stable _____

At Risk _____

High Risk _____

Related Event	% of Group of Diabetics Who Will Have the Event	Prevalence of Members with History of Events	Cost of Event	Cost if Have a History of Event
Cardiovascular				
Acute MI	_____	_____	_____	_____
Angina	_____	_____	_____	_____
Cerebrovascular				
Stroke	_____	_____	_____	_____
Transient ischemic attack	_____	_____	_____	_____
Nephropathy				
Microalbuminuria	_____	_____	_____	_____
Gross protienuria	_____	_____	_____	_____
ESRD	_____	_____	_____	_____
Retinopathy				
Background retinopathy	_____	_____	_____	_____
Macular edema	_____	_____	_____	_____
Proliferative diabetic retinopathy	_____	_____	_____	_____
Blindness	_____	_____	_____	_____
Neuropathy				
Symptomatic neuropathy	_____	_____	_____	_____
1st Lower extremity amputation	_____	_____	_____	_____
2nd Lower extremity amputation	_____	_____	_____	_____

Baseline medical cost per incident	**Cost**
Procedure	_____
Clinic visits (Diabetes 1 Gen Med)	_____
Medications (Diabetes 1 Gen Med)	_____

Exhibit 1 (*continued*)

Baseline medical cost per incident	Cost
Laboratory	_____
Equipment	_____
Blood glucose meter	_____
Blood testing strips	_____
Syringes	_____
Inpatient Days—Diabetes	_____
Inpatient Days—Gen Med Conditions	_____
Home health visits (Diabetes 1 Gen Med)	_____
Hospital Outpatient Encounter (DM 1 GM)	_____
Ambulatory Surgery (DM 1 GM)	_____
ER visits	_____
ER visits—Gen Med Conditions	_____

Graphically presented in Figure 2, this person-based model appears intuitive and elegant, but it is challenging to build. Future application developers will build modular components (or objects) that will act in a complementary way when combined with other components; these new combinations will in fact be greater than the sum of their parts.

Physician-Driven Designs and Patient Self-Monitoring. Today, physicians are largely left out of disease-management activities. The reasons are complicated and difficult to articulate well. Many believe that physicians will not or cannot contribute to the design of the disease-management program. Future disease-management programs will make the physician an active partner. The physician will build a program for an individual patient, hand it off to a disease manager for implementation, and then act as the moderator for the process.

Additionally, patients will be asked to monitor their own program and assume responsibility for their care by using an "owners' manual" for the body. Self-responsibility for timing laboratory tests and regular exams or for obtaining ongoing instructions will become a growing expectation, for instance.

Data Integration. Either data sources will increase and data formats will become standardized or the healthcare industry will be crushed under its own collective weight. Interestingly, self-reported data—data from patients— will take on a new meaning and be considered more valuable than ever. Nowhere in conventional medicine is there a repository for self-reported medication use, for example. Physicians, however, find this data useful when attempting to determine medication compliance and proper dosing schedules and frequency.

Figure 2. Person-Based Schematic

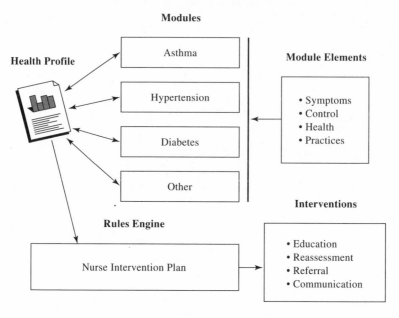

Data integration in its ultimate form will work in the background with expert systems to aid clinical judgment and the development of reasonable interventions. Medications, laboratory results, utilization rates, and self-reported data, when combined and applied to clinical logic, will form the basis of this new feature.

Let's use an asthma example to describe the possibilities. Medication records for patient X indicate that he is using 3.5 rescue inhalers per month (indicating an improper medication regime and poor symptom control); he has had two visits to the emergency room in the past six weeks; and he reports continued symptoms. The application would apply rules that produce an alert and suggested instructions for a plan of care. The physician uses the data and suggestions as a prompt to either follow or adjust the recommendation.

Increased Objective Data from Remote Sites. There is and there will continue to be a proliferation of remote downloadable monitoring devices.[15] These devices measure peak flow, blood glucose, weight, and blood pressure, and they collect survey data. The captured information is automatically downloaded to a central repository, then routed to a variety of sources for review and possible action.

These data will enter future systems by the "back door," will be evaluated, and, if necessary, will be acted on. The opportunities with these new technologies are endless, and they will be an important component in the not-so-distant future.

Figure 3. Multiple Users of a Disease-Management Database for a Cholesterol Test

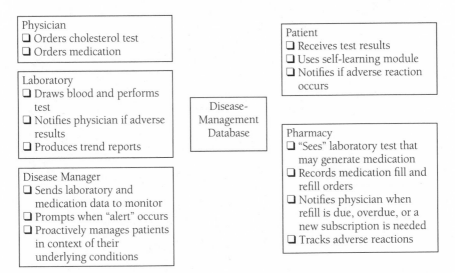

Physician
❑ Orders cholesterol test
❑ Orders medication

Laboratory
❑ Draws blood and performs test
❑ Notifies physician if adverse results
❑ Produces trend reports

Disease Manager
❑ Sends laboratory and medication data to monitor
❑ Prompts when "alert" occurs
❑ Proactively manages patients in context of their underlying conditions

Disease-Management Database

Patient
❑ Receives test results
❑ Uses self-learning module
❑ Notifies if adverse reaction occurs

Pharmacy
❑ "Sees" laboratory test that may generate medication
❑ Records medication fill and refill orders
❑ Notifies physician when refill is due, overdue, or a new subscription is needed
❑ Tracks adverse reactions

Multiple Ports of Entry. Next-generation disease-management programs will allow for multiple entry points into the program, most likely web-based. The application may look different to the physician, patient, disease manager, and payer. Communication within the program will be filtered by "the need to know" and expertise. See Figure 3 for a simple example using a cholesterol test.

Conclusion

Designing and implementing a disease-management program is difficult—so difficult that although many have tried, few have truly succeeded.[16] The nature of human responses to healthcare interventions adds an interesting dimension to the predictable world of application development. Combine unpredictable responses with the complexity of reimbursement systems and the political aspects of introducing another member to the healthcare team, and you get a tangled web.

The history of disease management indicates why disease management is a good idea and why it is happening at the right time. The state of healthcare today also necessitates an improved system of longitudinal care. And, finally, the technology exists to put the pieces of the puzzle together.

The next steps are ours: to make the correct early moves, measure our results, make corrections, then try again. Deming would be proud.

References

1. Marwick, C. "Another Health Care Idea: Disease Management." *Journal of the American Medical Association,* 1995, *274,* 1416–1417.
2. Epstein, R. S., and Sherwood, L. M. "From Outcomes Research to Disease Management: A Guide for the Perplexed." *Annals of Internal Medicine,* 1996, *124* (9), 832–837.
3. Hoffman, C. "Persons with Chronic Conditions: Their Prevalence and Costs." *Journal of the American Medical Association,* 1996, *276,* 1473–1479.
4. Huntington, J., and Connell, F. A. "For Every Dollar Spent—The Cost-Savings Argument for Prenatal Care." *New England Journal of Medicine,* 1994, *331,* 1303–1307.
5. Harris, J. M. "Disease Management: New Wine in New Bottles?" *Annals of Internal Medicine,* 1996, *124* (9), 832–837.
6. Zook, C. J., and Moore, F. D. "High-Cost Users of Medical Care." *New England Journal of Medicine,* 1980, *302,* 996–1002.
7. Rall, C. J., Munshi, A. D., and Stasior, D. S. "Disease Management and the Gastroenterologist." *Gastroenterology Clinics,* 1997, *26* (4), 874–894.
8. Brailer, D. J., and Dandrige, J. "Information Systems for Disease Management." In J. B. Couch (ed.), *The Physician's Guide to Disease Management.* Gaithersburg, Md.: Aspen, 1997.
9. Curtin, K., Hayes, D., Holland, C., and Katz, L. "Computer Generated Intervention for Asthma Population Care Management Objectives/Goals." *HMO Innovations Report,* 1998.
10. Miyashiro, R. "Catching Chameleons: Managing the Patient Identification in Evolving Health Care Systems." *Journal of Healthcare Information Management,* 1998, *12* (3) 53–62.
11. Califf, R., Vidaillet, R., and Goldman, L. "Managing the Patient with Advanced Heart Failure: Advanced Congestive Heart Failure: What Do Patients Want?" *Yearbook of Cardiology,* 1998, *135* (6), 153–157.
12. Burton, W., and Connerty, C. "Evaluation of a Worksite-Based Patient Education Intervention Targeted at Employees with Diabetes Mellitus." *Journal of Occupational and Environmental Medicine,* 1998, *40* (8), 702–706.
13. Pelletier, K. "Clinical and Cost Outcomes of Multifactorial, Cardiovascular Risk Management Interventions in Worksites: A Comprehensive Review and Analysis." *Journal of Occupational and Environmental Medicine,* 1997, *39* (12) 1154–1169.
14. Bennett, P. "Care Coordination in an Academic Medical Center." *Nursing Case Management,* 1997, *2* (2), 75–82.
15. Grigsby, J., and others. "Effects and Effectiveness of Telemedicine." *Health Care Financing Review,* 1995, *17,* 27–34.
16. "Disease Management Programs: Benchmarking Costs, Savings, ROI." *Health Benchmarks,* 1998, *5* (8), 117–119.

About the Authors

Rufus S. Howe, F.N.P., is vice president for product integration at Access Health Inc., Broomfield, Colorado.

Michael B. Terpening is senior director of systems analysis at Access Health Inc., Broomfield, Colorado.

Sandeep Wadhwa, M.D., M.B.A., is a fellow in the Division of Geriatrics and General Internal Medicine, University of Pennsylvania Hospital, Philadelphia.

Clinical Decision Support in Ambulatory Care: Tools, Trials, and Tribulations

J. Marc Overhage, M.D., Ph.D.; William M. Tierney, M.D.; Clement J. McDonald, M.D.

Any doctor who can be replaced by a computer deserves to be.
—Howard Bleich[1]

Improvements in the care process and consequent improvements in patient outcomes should be expected from the use of clinical decision support systems (CDSS) because physicians control 75 percent of all healthcare costs, bear primary responsibility for quality, and are the focal point for information collection. They perform these functions in a difficult environment; they must synthesize medical knowledge with the patient's data and integrate the impact of the costs and benefits of diagnostic and treatment options to decide on an intended course of action (Figure 1). Carrying out these intentions may be hindered by a variety of barriers. Competing priorities, such as dealing with the patient's presenting symptoms (usually the primary task of an outpatient encounter), distract attention from secondary tasks such as delivering preventive care or managing chronic diseases. A system for organizing, processing, and presenting relevant information at critical times may reduce physicians' mental workloads and direct attention to tasks that they might otherwise overlook.[2]

CDSS in outpatient order management can remind the clinician about what is true about the patient (previous abnormal test results, diagnoses) and what to do about it (suggested treatments, monitoring tests, screening, follow-up testing).[3] Managing information in an ambulatory setting requires 33 to 50 percent of a clinician's time.[4][5] Despite this substantial investment in time, information needs often go unmet. Half of the time clinicians proceed without the missing knowledge, and when they do seek to obtain the knowledge, it is usually by asking a colleague.[6] The timely availability of electronic patient information could reduce the duplication of tests because multiple providers in multiple sites could obtain recent and prior results. Moreover,

Figure 1. A Simple but Useful Behavioral Model
for Clinical Decision Processes

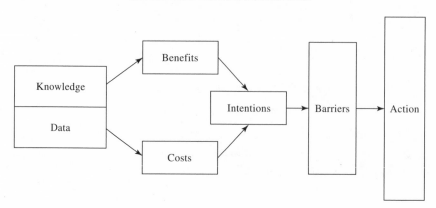

false positive results, and the subsequent tests needed to confirm or treat such results, could be reduced by targeting higher risk patients. Clinicians follow a variety of decision-making strategies,[7] including hypothesis testing,[8] scripts,[9] and heuristics,[10] rather than reasoned models of clinical decision making, such as Pauker's threshold model.[11] Information systems can help design complex models and can provide other information relevant to the clinical context (patient, setting, disease, test, drug).[12] The primary role of a CDSS is to bring precisely the right information to the clinician's attention in a highly useable format at exactly the right moment. Outpatient order management lends itself more to an interactive mode of clinical decision support (CDS), but it can have elements of both critiquing and consulting modes (complaining about a bad choice and suggesting good choices).

Prescriptions, diagnostic tests, nursing interventions, referrals, patient educational directions, diets, and nearly everything else a clinician directs to be done for a patient can be conceptualized as an order. Requirements for referral, patient activities, and order management in the outpatient setting have many similarities with those for inpatient settings but have some differences as well. Implementing advice from CDSS may be more difficult in outpatient settings because of timing. Unless the CDSS is used directly at the point of care, the practitioner must relay changes in plans that result from feedback from CDSS to the patient, which can be much harder in an outpatient than in an inpatient setting. In the inpatient setting, the provider often goes ahead and orders tests or other interventions, relying on the nursing or other ancillary staff to inform the patient. Timing of actions is often tied more to events (on the next visit) than to explicit time frames (in the morning). The scope of care delivered in the outpatient setting is broader and covers more issues, so there is more need for a decision-support system but also more risk that the provider will be overwhelmed by a large volume of feedback. There are also many more providers of services, such as laboratories, pharmacies, and health plans, to deal with in the outpatient setting.

Historical Overview of Outpatient Order Management

Some of the earliest outpatient CDSS were diagnostic, such as de Dombal's Leeds Abdominal Pain System.[13] The most widely available and most intensively studied CDSS in outpatient settings, however, are based on reminders to clinicians to perform preventive care. These systems are easier to implement because they do not require the clinician to interact directly with the system; instead, feedback can be delivered as printed reminders. Data in these systems were often originally captured from ancillary systems or from forms completed by the providers. Implementing more sophisticated interactions, including those necessary to recommend specific therapies, requires the major step of getting the provider to enter information and receive feedback directly from the CDSS. Depending on the data the clinician is entering, various kinds of decision support (drugs-allergy, drug-drug, drug-diagnosis information; screening; diagnosis monitoring; follow-up of treatments and tests; Evaluation and Management coding; appropriate drugs, tests, and nursing interventions) can be implemented.

Standards and Methods for Implementation of Outpatient Order Management

All CDSS can be thought of as having a knowledge base that is operated on by some kind of reasoning process, using patient-specific data, in order to provide feedback to the provider. Probably the most challenging aspect of implementing a CDSS is ensuring that the necessary data are available and valid. Lack of good data is one of the major barriers to use of diagnostic systems, for example. It is difficult to capture data because it comes from many places (many laboratories, mammograms, multiple providers writing prescriptions), and some data, such as fundoscopic or breast examinations, are not available in any ancillary system. Fortunately, standards for transmitting data among clinical systems—for example, Health Level Seven (HL7)[14] and Digital Imaging and Communications in Medicine (DICOM)[15]—and for coding data—for example, Logical Observation Identifier Names and Codes (LOINC)[16 17] and Systematized Nomenclature of Human Medicine-Reference Technology[18]—are evolving. Knowledge bases can be represented using several methods, but none has achieved wide enough application or solved data-access problems well enough to result in interchangeable, widely used knowledge bases. In addition, the content of knowledge bases must be specific to the outpatient environment. Conditional probabilities differ in inpatient and outpatient settings. Even in outpatient settings results may vary greatly. de Dombal's abdominal-pain system did not perform as well in other settings as it did in the original setting in Leeds.[19] [20] A variety of reasoning methods can also be applied to these knowledge bases, but only procedural systems have achieved widespread use.

Critical Functionality of Outpatient Order Management

Most of the evidence for improvements in the process and outcomes of medical care comes from CDSS that are integrated with a clinical-information system, or have access to a data suppository as Shortliffe has suggested[21] and integrate with clinical workflow.[22] [23] [24] [25] In addition, the care environment must be organized to facilitate evaluation of the reminders.[26]

A number of critical issues must be considered when developing feedback for CDSS.[27] *Speed* is always essential for clinician acceptance of an information system. A CDSS cannot introduce significant delays into the clinician's workflow. One way to satisfying this requirement is to precompute the feedback and then incrementally modify it at the time of clinical interaction as data are updated.

CDSS that are *active* have generally been more successful than passive systems.[28] Active systems deliver feedback, while passive systems require the provider to recognize that advice might be available and then to ask for it. Some systems take a middle ground, identifying feedback that is appropriate as soon as data are available but delivering the feedback when providers might be ready to receive it, such as the next time they are reviewing data for a specific patient.

Reminders must be *actionable*—that is, physicians must be able to take some action as a result of the reminder. Simply reminding them about facts that they can't do anything about will only frustrate them and will result in their paying less attention to reminders they get in the future. In addition, the action suggested by the reminder must fall *within the physician's domain of responsibility*. Reminding physicians responsible for a patient's care during an inpatient stay was largely ineffective when the physician was not the patient's primary-care provider. Although the physicians generally reported they would like preventive care delivered to their patients while hospitalized under another physician's care, they did not feel it appropriate to deliver preventive care to the patients they were caring for in the hospital for whom they were not the primary-care provider.[29]

Full sentences and correct grammar are less important than making good use of the available "advertising space" for reminders. The temptation is to create carefully worded, well-developed arguments, including detailed patient data, to support the reminder. Such an approach will generally fail because the physician will not invest the energy to read and understand a message that consists of several sentences. We have had greater success from crafting *terse, targeted text*. A reminder to treat a patient with diabetes and hypertension with an angiotensin-converting enzyme (ACE) inhibitor, for example, might be "treat with ACE inhibitor because of diabetes and HTN" followed by a suggested order for a specific ACE inhibitor at a reasonable dosage. The reminder is specific to the patient and conveys the underlying rationale but presumes that the physician will recognize the connection. A more detailed explanatory version of the reminder will usually be available as well.

The examples above illustrate another characteristic of successful reminders: they must be *patient-specific*. General reminders to treat patients with diabetes and hypertension with ACE inhibitors will not be as successful as reminders that concern a specific patient. First, a generic reminder forces physicians to do more mental work. They must remember that a reminder exists and then realize that it might apply to a specific patient. Second, physicians may not realize that a patient has one of the underlying conditions. Elevated blood pressures are commonly missed, and hypertension goes untreated, for example. Finally, important reminders will not be noticed if every generic reminder that might apply is generated for each patient.

Although reminders don't always have to be correct, they must be *correct about one-third of the time* for the physician to retain confidence in the system that generates them. To achieve this goal, the *sensitivity and specificity* of the logic that generates the reminders must be adjusted. One way to increase the specificity of reminders and at the same time limit the number of reminders the physician receives is to choose the extreme suggested limits. Inappropriate reminders are tolerated only because the physician acts as a filter to prevent inappropriate actions from being taken.

Reminder quality is limited by the quality of the data on which the reminders are based. Developers must have an acute *awareness of the content and limitations of the database* used to generate the reminders. Reminders about immunizations, for example, that come from a database that does not capture immunizations will be excessive and inappropriate.

The maximum effect on physician behavior is seen when reminders are delivered at the *point of care*. In a randomized trial, a reminder delivered after the patient encounter was not as effective as the same reminder delivered at the time of the encounter.[30] The difference in effect is likely due to differences in the barriers that prevent transforming the reminder into action. Physicians are more likely to take action if the patient is present. Reminders to obtain blood tests, collect information for a patient, start new therapies, or educate the patient are all more difficult to follow when the patient must be contacted outside an encounter. Forcing physicians to respond to reminders has been demonstrated to increase compliance for house physicians but not for experienced internists.[2]

Careful attention to details such as these is required if reminders are to affect physician behavior. Even small perturbations in the environment can nullify the effect of reminders. A transient delay in capturing mammogram results, for example, severely eroded provider confidence in reminders for mammography in a system in which the reminders had been appropriate for many years.[31] Physician memories for benefits are short, but they are long for mistakes or inconvenience.

Impact of Outpatient Order Management

Almost 60 percent of randomized clinical trials of CDSS have been performed in primary-care outpatient settings, with the remainder equally divided between specialty outpatient and inpatient settings.[28] Several systematic reviews summarize many of the studies of CDS in outpatient settings.[28 32 33 34] The most commonly tested effects included cancer-screening compliance rates,[35 36] vaccination rates,[37 38 39 40] blood-pressure measurements,[41 42 43] use of laboratory tests[38 44 45 46 47] prenatal-screening rates,[48 49] and medication-monitoring rates.[50 51 52]

In the early 1970s the Regenstrief Medical Record System, in addition to providing access to medical records, began helping clinicians by generating prospective, protocol-driven recommendations. These messages alerted clinicians to important clinical events in a patient's computerized medical record and reminded the physicians to take proper corrective action. The knowledge base consisted of simple rules. The system checked for evidence that monitoring tests had been ordered after certain drug therapies were initiated and for abnormal test results that, in combination with particular therapies, might suggest insufficient, excessive, or dangerous treatment. Whenever the system identified a patient who satisfied a condition in the rules, it printed a message on the encounter form for the responsible physician suggesting a specific action and the rational for the action. In a randomized, controlled trial[49], reminders increased compliance with suggested test orders from 11 to 36 percent and increased changes in drug therapy in response to a test result from 13 to 28 percent. In a subsequent study with 390 different protocols[45], physicians complied with reminders in 51 percent of cases when they received reminders. Their usual practice pattern resulted in compliance in 22 percent of the cases (when they were not receiving reminders). In addition, the crossover design of this study allowed McDonald to show that because the effects disappeared quickly when reminders were stopped, reminders did not teach the clinicians.

McDonald and his colleagues next created the CARE language to enable them to develop and maintain a larger number of protocols,[53] and they developed 1,491 rules. A study of these protocols in a randomized, controlled trial in a university-affiliated general internal-medicine practice showed that physicians performed the suggested actions in 47 percent of the cases but in only 29 percent of the cases when they were not reminded.

Similar results were obtained for specific protocols in studies carried out by others; the protocols included reminders for managing cases of streptococcal pharyngitis and for following up patients with diastolic hypertension at Harvard Community Health Plan,[54 55] reminders for cervical-cancer screening in a family-medicine practice,[56] and reminders for cancer screening in a private practice.[57] The rules in these early studies were simple, reinforcing the concept that the providers needed assistance in identifying conditions that required their attention.

Rising healthcare costs is an area of concern. Diagnostic tests account for a large share of total healthcare expenditures, and critics charge that they appear to have little effect on treatment.[58 59 60] Physicians are often unaware of the costs of these diagnostic tests. Further, they seldom know the probability of a positive test result.[61 62] They have no clear plan for using a test result to inform their therapeutic decisions. Interventions to reduce inefficient use of diagnostic tests have been reported,[63 64 65 66] but these interventions were either cost- or labor-intensive, and institutions could not maintain them in the long term.

Several studies of clinicians interacting with an early clinical workstation that incorporated simple CDSS demonstrated that CDSS can be a sustainable, affordable intervention for achieving these aims. Displaying the last result and how long ago it was obtained for eight selected diagnostic tests decreased average test charges per visit by 13 percent, reflecting 8.5 percent fewer test orders for study patients. Testing rates during the interactive period for both study and control patients decreased by 16.8 and 10.9 percent from the preintervention period, suggesting that experience during study visits influenced test ordering. The exposure to the display of previous data may have stimulated physicians to review all patients' flowcharts more carefully than they had in the past. Orders for the tests included in the study increased by 10.6 percent after the intervention period, a finding that suggests that the decline during the intervention (which was significantly higher for study patients) was not due solely to temporal trends.[65] Similar results were obtained in the second intervention, in which the probability that the test would be positive for the abnormality under investigation was displayed. During the six-month controlled trial, charges were 8.8 percent lower for study patients. Displaying the charge for the test being ordered and the total charges for tests ordered that day in the third intervention had the largest effects. During the six-month intervention period, physicians in the study group ordered 14 percent fewer tests per visit than the control-group physicians did, resulting in 13 percent lower charges. There were no differences in the number of hospitalizations, emergency-room visits, or visits to an outpatient clinic during the six months following the intervention, indicating that quality had not been adversely effected.

These studies have shown that different types of computer assistance could significantly reduce the costs of diagnostic tests without any reduction in the quality of care.[59 60 65] The study investigators believe that the intervention reduced test ordering because physicians made better decisions when presented with concise displays of relevant patient information at the time the test was being ordered.[65]

As ambulatory-care information systems with order-entry components become more common, integrated decision-support capabilities like these can make physicians more aware of the relative costs and benefits of diagnostic testing. Presenting relevant information at the right time is an easy task for a computer system when its patient database contains both clinical and administrative data. The cost and effort associated with the additional programming are low, and these CDSS might help to control increases in healthcare costs.

Displaying fully formed orders for clinicians as a consequence of their entering other orders or consequent orders markedly increased the frequency with which appropriate follow-up tests or adjunct medications were ordered.[59] These orders were offered for review when the "trigger" orders were entered, a time when physicians were receptive to feedback related to the "trigger" order. In addition, because the orders were fully formed, completing the order required minimal effort.

To date, little evidence suggests that diagnostic decision-support systems are useful. A systematic review[60] revealed that only one in five studies indicated an improvement in outcomes; these systems provided the correct diagnosis 52 to 71 percent of the time and included only half the relevant diagnoses.[65]

Future Trends for Outpatient Order Management

The experience to date shows not only that physicians will use computer workstations but that they will respond to interventions during online order writing to lower costs and improve the quality of care. Physicians respond to feedback that is delivered in a timely manner, represents acceptable clinical decisions, and is patient- and problem-specific. Inserting electronic information management into the processes of care presents an opportunity to provide generic and problem-specific information at the very moment physicians are making clinical decisions. For example, a drug-interaction alert needs to be integrated both with the relevant data sources (medical record containing coded data for drug allergies, laboratory results, and existing medication) and with a computer-based prescribing system, so that it can be issued automatically and will reach the person who needs to take action. Providers can be encouraged both to increase the ordering of underused tests (for example, for preventive care or monitoring of inpatient drug therapy) and to reduce the ordering of overused tests.

Once some of the more immediate barriers are overcome, prioritizing and filtering CDSS feedback to focus the clinician's attention will become more important. As the quantity of data available increases and medical knowledge evolves, the amount of feedback the provider receives increases dramatically, leading to information overload and an ineffective CDSS. Some early adopters of CDSS are already confronting this issue as their knowledge bases grow. Matching the kind of advice and its presentation closely with users' requirements, including their level of knowledge and the kinds of dilemmas they routinely face, is essential. Otherwise, providers may be overwhelmed with alerts and reminders that they find incomprehensible or too obvious to merit their attention. Techniques such as belief networks are now being explored as one way to determine which feedback is most important to deliver at a given point in time.

The medical literature contains guidelines that range from simple, unambiguous, and easily implemented rules to large, unsubstantiated opinions of "expert" committees.[67] Every effort should be made to derive as much as possible of the systems knowledge base from rigorous evidence and to avoid the opinions of individual experts.[68] Even carefully researched guidelines developed using rigorous methods lack the specificity required for direct use in a CDSS.[69] The challenges confronted in developing such content are evident from examination of efforts to integrate a broad spectrum of guidelines into a CDSS such as the Prodigy project in Great Britain.[70] This integration has been achieved on at least one occasion.[71]

There are no legal precedents on which to base a resolution of the key issue: negligence law and strict liability principles will be applied.[72] Negligence law requires a product to meet reasonable expectations for safety, while strict liability requires that a product not be harmful. A related question is clinicians' liability if they rely on feedback from a CDSS in their decision making or if they do not use a CDSS that has become the community standard of care. Current Federal Drug Administration policy is that CDSS are not subject to regulation because a trained practitioner is receiving and evaluating the feedback.[73]

Finally, CDSS require ongoing rigorous evaluation, including assessment of their structure, functions (such as accuracy, time to give advice), and impact on the users' decisions and the clinical problem.[74] [75] Rigorous evaluation of CDSS are important, just as it is for any other expensive healthcare technology, because these systems have the potential for harm as well as for improving the quality and controlling the cost of care.[73] [76]

References

1. Bleich, H. L., and others. "Clinical Computing in a Teaching Hospital." *New England Journal of Medicine,* 1985, *3312,* 756–764.
2. Powsner, S. M., Wyatt, J. C., and Wright, P. "Medical Records: Opportunities and Challenges of Computerisation." *Lancet,* 1998, *352,* 1617–1622.
3. Healthfield, H. A., and Wyatt, J. C. "Philosophies for the Design and Development of Clinical Decision Support Systems." *Methods of Information in Medicine,* 1993, *32,* 1–8.
4. Wipf, J. E., Fihn, S. D., Callahan, C. M., and Phillips, C. M. "How Residents Spend Their Time in Clinic and the Effects of Clerical Support." *Journal of General Internal Medicine,* 1994, *9,* 694–696.
5. Smith, D. M, Martin, D. K., Langefeld, C. D., Miller, M. E., and Freedman, J. A. "Primary Care Physician Productivity: The Physician Factor." *Journal of General Internal Medicine,* 1995, *10,* 495–503.
6. Coull, D., Uman, G., and Manning, P. "Information Needs of Office Practices: Are They Being Met?" *Annals of Internal Medicine,* 1985, *3,* 596–599.
7. Wyatt, J. "Use and Sources of Medical Knowledge." *Lancet,* 1991, *338,* 1368–1373.

8. Elstern, A. S., Shulman, L. S., and Sprafka, S. A. *Medical Problem Solving.* Cambridge, Mass.: Harvard University Press, 1978.
9. Patel, V., Evans, D., and Green, G. "Biomedical Knowledge and Clinical Reasoning." In D. Evans and V. Patel (eds.), *Cognitive Science in Medicine.* Cambridge, Mass.: MIT Press, 1986.
10. McDonald, C. J. "Medical Heuristics: The Silent Adjudicators of Clinical Practice." *Annals of Internal Medicine,* 1996, *124* (1, pt. 1), 56–62.
11. Pauker, S. G., and Kassirer, J. P. "The Threshold Approach to Clinical Decision Making." *New England Journal of Medicine,* 1980, *302,* 1109–1117.
12. McDonald, C. J., Overhage, J. M., Tierney, W. M., Abernathy, G. R., and Dexter, P. R. "The Promise of Computerized Feedback Systems for Diabetes Care." *Annals of Internal Medicine,* 1996, *124,* 170–174.
13. de Dombal, F. T., Leaper, D. J., Staniland, J. R., McCann, A. P., and Horrocks, J. C. "Computer Aided Diagnosis of Acute Abdominal Pain." *British Medical Journal,* 1972, *1,* 376–380.
14. Health Level Seven. *An Application Protocol for Electronic Data Exchange in Healthcare Environments, Version 2.3.* Ann Arbor, Mich.: Health Level Seven, 1997.
15. Digital Imaging and Communications in Medicine. *The ACR NEMA DICOM Standard.* Publication PS3.1 PS3.12. Rosslyn, Va.; National Electrical Manufacturers Association, 1995.
16. Huff, S. M., and others. "Development of the Logical Observation Identifier Names and Codes (LOINC) Vocabulary." *Journal of the American Medical Informatics Association,* 1998, *5* (3), 276–292.
17. Forrey, A. W., and others. "The Logical Observation Identifier Names and Codes (LOINC) Database: A Public Use Set of Codes and Names for Electronic Reporting of Clinical Laboratory Test Results." *Clinical Chemistry,* 1996, *2,* 81–90.
18. Spackman, K. A., Campbell, K. E., and Cote, R. A. "SNOMED RT: A Reference Terminology for Health Care." *AMIA Fall Symposium Proceedings, Journal of the American Medical Informatics Association Symposium Supplement,* October 25, 1997, pp. 640–644.
19. Sutton, G. C. "Computers in Medicine: How Accurate Is Computer Aided Diagnosis?" *Lancet,* 1989, *2,* 905–908.
20. Paterson Brown, S., and others. "Clinical Decision Making and Laparascopy Versus Computer Prediction in the Management of the Acute Abdomen." *British Journal of Surgery,* 1989, *76,* 1011–1013.
21. Shortliffe, E. H. "Knowledge-Based Systems in Medicine." *Proceedings of Medical Informatics in Europe,* 1991, 5–9.
22. McDonald, C. J., Tierney, W. M., Martin, D. K., and Overhage, J. M. "The Regenstrief Medical Record System: 20 Years of Experience in Hospitals, Clinics and Neighborhood Health Centers." *MD Computing,* 1992, *9* (4), 206–217.
23. Safran, C., and others. "Computer-Based Support for Clinical Decision Making." *MD Computing,* 1990, *7,* 319–322.
24. Hammond, W. E. "TMR—A profile of an Electronic Patient Record." *Proceedings of MedInfo,* 1992, *1,* 730–735.
25. Kuperman, G. J., Gardner, R. M., and Pryor, T. A. *HELP: A Dynamic Hospital Information System.* New York: Springer-Verlag, 1991.
26. Tierney, W. M., Miller, M. E., Hui, S. L., and McDonald, C. J. "Practice Randomization and Clinical Research: The Indiana Experience." *Medical Care,* 1991, *29* (supplement), JS57–JS64.
27. Overhage, J. M. "Secrets of the Reminder Gurus: How to Change Physician Behavior with Information." Toward an Electronic Patient Record, 13th Annual Symposium, 1997.
28. Balas, E. A., Austin, S. M., Mitchell, J. A., and Wigman, E., "The Clinical Value of Computerized Information Services: A Review of 98 Randomized Clinical Trials." *Archives of Family Medicine,* 1996, *5,* 271–278.
29. Overhage, J. M., Tierney, W. M., and McDonald, C. J. "Computer Reminders to Implement Preventive Care Guidelines for Hospital Inpatients." *Archives of Internal Medicine,* 1996, *156,* 1551–1556.

30. Tierney, W. M., Hui, S. L., and McDonald, C. J. "Delayed Feedback of Physician Performance Versus Immediate Reminders to Perform Preventive Care: Effects on Physician Compliance." *Medical Care,* 1986, *24,* 659–666.
31. Banks, N. J., and others. "Implementation and Evaluation of a Computerized Reminder System in Ambulatory Care." *Proceedings of the Annual Symposium on Computer Applications in Medical Care,* 1998, *12,* 753-757.
32. Sullivan, F., and Mitchell, E. "Has General Practitioner Computing Made a Difference to Patient Care? A Systematic Review of Published Reports." *British Medical Journal,* 1995, *311,* 848–852.
33. Johnston, M. E., Langton, K. B., Hayes, B., and Mathieu, A. "Effects of Computer-Based Clinical Decision Support Systems on Clinician Performance and Patient Outcome: A Critical Appraisal of Research." *Annals of Internal Medicine,* 1994, *120,* 135–142.
34. Haynes, R. B., and Walker, C. J. "Computer-Aided Quality Assurance. A Critical Appraisal." *Archives of Internal Medicine,* 1987, *147,* 1297–1301.
35. Banks, N. J., and others. "Implementation and Evaluation of a Computerized Reminder System in Ambulatory Care." *Proceedings of the Annual Symposium on Computer Applications in Medical Care,* 2, 753–757.
36. Chambers, C. V., and others. "Microcomputer-Generated Reminders: Improving the Compliance of Primary Care Physicians with Mammography Screening Guidelines." *Journal of Family Practice,* 1989, *3,* 273–280.
37. Brimberry, R. "Vaccination of High-Risk Patients for Influenza: A Comparison of Telephone and Mail Reminder Methods." *Journal of Family Practice,* 1988, *26,* 397–400.
38. McDonald, C. J., and others. "Reminders to Physicians from an Introspective Computer Medical Record: A 2-Year Randomized Trial." *Annals of Internal Medicine,* 1984, *100,* 130–138.
39. Ornstein, S. M., Garr, D. R., Jenkins, R. G., Rust, P. F, and Arnon, A. "Computer-Generated Physician and Patient Reminders: Tools to Improve Population Adherence to Selected Preventive Services." *Journal of Family Practice,* 1991, *32,* 82–90.
40. Soljak, M. A., and Handford, S. "Early Results from the Northland Immunisation Register." *New Zealand Medical Journal,* 1987, *100,* 244–246.
41. Barnett, G. O., Winickoff, R. N., Morgan, M. M., and Zielstorff, R. D. "A Computer-Based Monitoring System for Follow-Up of Elevated Blood Pressure." *Medical Care,* 1983, *21,* 400–409.
42. Burling, T. A., and others. "Computerized Smoking Cessation Program for the Worksite: Treatment Outcome and Feasibility." *Journal of Consulting and Clinical Psychology,* 1989, *5,* 619–622.
43. Rogers, J. L., Haring, O. M., and Goetz, J. P. "Changes in Patient Attitudes Following the Implementation of a Medical Information System." *QRB Quality Review Bulletin,* Mar. 10, 1984, pp. 65–74.
44. Rogers, J. L., Haring, O. M., and Watson, R. A. "Automating the Medical Record: Emerging Issues." *Proceedings of the Annual Symposium on Computer Applications in Medical Care,* 1979, *3,* 255–263.
45. Berwick, D. M., and Coltin, K. L. "Feedback Reduces Test Use in a Health Maintenance Organization." *Journal of the American Medical Association,* 1986, *255,* 1450–1454.
46. McDonald, C. J. "Protocol-Based Computer Reminders, the Quality of Care and the Non-perfectibility of Man." *New England Journal of Medicine,* 1976, *295,* 1351–1355.
47. McDonald, C. J., Wilson, G. A., and McCabe, G. P. "Physician Response to Computer Reminders." *Journal of the American Medical Association,* 1980, *244,* 1579–1581.
48. Morgan, M., Studney, D. R., Barnett, G. O., and Winickoff, R. N. "Computerized Concurrent Review of Prenatal Care." *QRB Quality Review Bulletin,* Sept. 4, 1978, pp. 33–36.
49. Hofmeyr, G. J., Pattinson, R., Buckley, D., Jennings, J., and Redman, C. W. "Umbilical Artery Resistance Index as a Screening Test for Fetal Well-Being: Randomized Feasibility Study." *Obstetrics and Gynecology,* 1991, *78,* 359–362.

50. McDonald, C. J. "Use of Computer to Detect and Respond to Clinical Events: Its Effect on Clinician Behavior." *Annals of Internal Medicine,* 1976, *84,* 162–167.

51. Schrezenmeir, J., Achterberg, H., and Bergeler, J., "Controlled Study on the Use of Hand-Held Insulin Dosage Computers Enabling Conversion to and Optimizing of Meal-Related Insulin Therapy Regimens." *Life Support Systems,* 1985, *3* (supplement), 561–567.

52. White, K. S., Lindsay, A., Pryor, T. A., Brown, W. F., and Walsh, K. "Application of a Computerized Medical Decision-Making Process to the Problem of Digoxin Intoxication." *Journal of the American College of Cardiology,* 1984, *4,* 571–576.

53. McDonald, C. J. *Action-Oriented Decisions in Ambulatory Medicine.* St. Louis, Mo.: Mosby-Year Book, 1981.

54. Barnett, G. O., Winickoff, R. N., Dorsey, J. L., Morgan, M. M., and Lurie, R. S. "Quality Assurance Through Automated Monitoring and Concurrent Feedback Using a Computer-Based Medical Information System." *Medical Care,* 1978, *16,* 961–970.

55. McDowell, I., Newell, C., and Rosser, W. "Computerized Reminders to Encourage Cervical Screening in Family Practice." *Journal of Family Practice,* 1989, *28,* 420–424.

56. McPhee, S. J., Bird, J. A., Fordham, D., Rodnick, J. E., and Osorn, E. H. "Promoting Cancer Prevention Activities by Primary Care Physicians." *Journal of the American Medical Association,* 1991, *266,* 538–544.

57. Olsen, D. M., Kane, R. L., and Proctor, P. H. "A Controlled Trial of Multiphasic Screening." *New England Journal of Medicine,* 1976, *294,* 925–930.

58. Shapiro, M. F., Hatch, R. L., and Greenfield, S. "Cost Containment and Labor-Intensive Tests: The Case of the Leukocyte Differential Count." *Journal of the American Medical Association,* 1984, *252,* 231–234.

59. Hubbel, F. A., Greenfield, S., Tyler, J. L., Chetty, K., and Wyle, F. A. "The Impact of Routine Admission Chest X-Ray Films on Patient Care." *New England Journal of Medicine,* 1985, *312,* 209–212.

60. Tierney, W. M., McDonald, C. J., Hui, S. L., and Martin, D. K. "Computerized Predictions of Abnormal Test Results." *Journal of the American Medical Association,* 1988, *259,* 1194–1198.

61. Tierney, W. M., Miller, M. E., and McDonald, C. J. "The Effects on Test Ordering of Informing Physicians of the Charges for Outpatient Diagnostic Tests." *New England Journal of Medicine,* 1990, *322,* 1499–1504.

62. Rhyne, R. L., and Gehlbach, S. H. "Effects of an Educational Feedback Strategy on Physician Utilization of Thyroid Function Panels." *Journal of Family Practice,* 1979, *8,* 1003–1007.

63. Williams, S. V., and Eisenberg, J. M. "A Controlled Trial to Decrease the Unnecessary Use of Diagnostic Tests." *Journal of General Internal Medicine,* 1986, *1,* 8–13.

64. Wong, E. T., McCarron, M. M., and Shaw, S. T., Jr. "Ordering of Laboratory Tests in a Teaching Hospital: Can It Be Improved?" *Journal of the American Medical Association,* 1983, *249,* 3076–3080.

65. Haynes, R. B., Davis, D. A., McCibbon, A., and Tugwell, P. "A Critical Appraisal of the Efficacy of Continuing Medical Education." *Journal of the American Medical Association,* 1984, *251,* 61–64.

66. Tierney, W. M., McDonald, C. J., Martin, D. K., Hui, S. L., and Rogers, M. P. "Computerized Display of Past Test Results." *Annals of Internal Medicine,* 1987, *107,* 569–574.

67. McDonald, C. J., and Overhage, J. M. "Guidelines You Can Follow and Trust: An Ideal and an Example." *Journal of the American Medical Association,* 1994, *271,* 872–873.

68. Antman, E. M., Lau, J., Kupelnick, B., Mosteller, F., and Chalmers, T. C. "A Comparison of Results of Meta-Analyses of Randomized Control Trials and Recommendations of Clinical Experts." *Journal of the American Medical Association,* 1992, *268,* 240–248.

69. Tierney, W. M., Overhage, J. M., Takesue, B. Y., Harris, L. E., Murray, M. D., Vargo, D. L., and McDonald, C. J. "Computerizing Guidelines to Improve Care and Patient Outcomes." *Journal of the American Medical Informatics Association,* 1995, *2,* 316–322.

70. Purves, I. *PRODIGY Interim Report.* Newcastle upon Tyne: Sowerby Unit for Primary Care Informatics, University of Newcastle, 1996.
71. Holbrooke, A., Langton, K., Haynes, R. B., Mathieu, A., and Cowan, S. "PREOP: Development of an Evidence-Based Expert System to Assist with Preoperative Assessments." In P. Clayton (ed.), *Proceedings of the 15th Annual Symposium on Computer Applications in Medical Care.* New York: McGraw-Hill, 1991.
72. Miller, R. A., Schaffner, K., and Meisal, A. "Ethical and Legal Issues Related to the Use of Computer Programs in Clinical Medicine." *Annals of Internal Medicine,* 1985, *102,* 529–537.
73. Young, F. "Validation of Medical Software: Present Policy at the Food and Drug Administration." *Annals of Internal Medicine,* 1987, *106,* 628.
74. Wyatt, J., and Spiegelhalter, D. "Evaluating Medical Expert Systems: What to Test and How?" *Medical Informatics,* 1990, *15,* 205–217.
75. Wyatt, J., and Spiegelhalter, D. "Field Trials of Medical Decision-Aids: Potential Problems and Solutions." In P. Clayton (ed.), *Proceedings of the 15th Annual Symposium on Computer Applications in Medical Care.* New York: McGraw-Hill, 1991.
76. Tierney, W. M., and McDonald, C. J. "Testing Informatics Innovations: The Value of Negative Trials." *Journal of the American Medical Informatics Association,* 1996, *3,* 358–359.

About the Authors

J. Marc Overhage, M.D., Ph.D., is an investigator with the Regenstrief Institute and assistant professor of medicine at the Indiana University School of Medicine, Indianapolis.

William M. Tierney, M.D., is associate professor of medicine at the Regenstrief Institute Indiana University Medical Center.

Clement J. McDonald, M.D., is associate professor of medicine at the Regenstrief Institute Indiana University Medical Center.

Clinical Decision Support for Hospital and Critical Care

Gilad J. Kuperman, M.D., Ph.D.; Dean F. Sittig, Ph.D.;
M. Michael Shabot, M.D., FACS, FCCM, FACMI

The acute- and critical-care medical settings are distinguished from other medical settings in three ways: patients in these settings are the most ill, decisions made by caregivers carry the greatest short-term consequences, and many more data are involved in decision making. Caregivers who work in these settings face different challenges than do clinicians who work in such settings as outpatient clinics, nursing homes, and emergency rooms. This article presents an overview of applications of clinical decision support systems (CDSS) that have been developed to aid caregivers as they work in these settings. The article focuses on knowledge-based decision support, although other kinds of decision support are discussed. The article mentions only cursorily decision support in the ordering process because this topic is covered elsewhere in this volume.

Historical Overview

CDSS in the hospital and acute-care settings have a long and distinguished history. In 1961, Warner[1] used site-specific pressure data obtained during cardiac catheterization (a new technique at that time) and Bayesian probabilistic techniques developed by Ledley and Lusted[2] to demonstrate that computers could diagnose congenital heart disease as well as expert clinicians. Since then, the use of computers to provide automated CDSS has been an active and diverse area of research and development.

Several researchers have continued to explore the use of computers to assist with diagnosis. Examples of such efforts are Mycin,[3] Internist-1,[4] DXplain,[5] and Iliad.[6] Several vexing issues, including the best way to represent knowledge in the computer, how to make decisions in the face of missing data, and how to reason when uncertainty is present, have been explored in the course of these projects.[7,8] Such potential solutions as procedural knowledge representation and the use of rules, statistics, Bayesian belief networks, and neural networks have been examined for their ability to support the diagnostic process. No single computer program is robust enough yet to match expert clinicians' diagnostic skills; however much has been learned about the abilities and limitations of such programs. Many of the aforementioned programs currently are in use in an educational mode.

Clinical-information systems began to be developed in the late 1960s. Since then, several institutions have explored the various ways in which decision-support features can be incorporated into clinical applications. The distinguishing feature of these applications is the presence of a clinical database that can be used to generate patient-specific suggestions without the need for data to be reentered. Over the years, several different kinds of data have been incorporated into the patient database, and their incorporation has led to diverse kinds of CDSS. Today, clinical patient databases include demographic and administrative data, laboratory results, medication data (both inpatient and outpatient), allergy data, radiology results, structured and unstructured clinical-documentation data (from physicians, nurses, and other clinicians), data from several different devices in intensive-care units (ICUs) (monitors, ventilators, intravenous pumps), and physician orders. The functions that make use of all these data are discussed in the section on critical functionality below.

Technology has had an important impact on CDSS. Computing platforms through the 1980s were mainly mainframe-based. The advent of personal computers (with improved screen graphics), local-area networks, and client-server architectures in the 1990s led to improved clinical usability. Improved screen graphics are the basis for new user interfaces that enable a much higher level of interaction with clinicians. New user interfaces have improved results-review applications, have enabled clinical data-entry applications such as physician order entry, and permit waveform data (electrocardiograms, monitored data in the ICU) to be displayed. Client-server architectures permit CD-ROM-based knowledge bases to be incorporated into clinical-information systems. More recently, the Internet has provided a powerful new computing platform. Internet-based applications can be widely distributed and easily maintained and offer several new opportunities for information distribution and decision support. Although the Internet provides many advantages, many problems that were difficult to resolve in mainframe environments remain difficult to resolve with newer technologies. For example, an automated infusion system for titration of dopamine for patients in hemodynamic crisis has been an unattainable goal thus far; the advent of the Internet will not make this problem easier to solve.

Current research questions in CDSS include how best to represent clinical disease-management guidelines in the computer and how to integrate their use into routine clinical care. Other current work includes development of enabling technologies such as natural language processing (NLP) software— that is, software that extracts coded findings from narrative text documents (reports of chest x-rays, dictated notes). Such documents represent a rich source of coded findings if NLP software can be successful.[9]

The new graphical user interfaces such as those in the Windows 95 and Internet browser environments are gaining wider acceptance. Software using these interfaces allows more data to be collected and more decision support to be provided. Speech-recognition software is another interface technology that holds promise for capturing (free text) data; however, as of this writing the technology is still somewhat cumbersome and is not in widespread use.

The development of dictionaries and data models to represent clinical concepts has provided the nontrivial and critical underpinning of all decision-support activities. The creation of terms for such clinical items as problem lists, medication lists, allergies, radiology examinations, laboratory tests, symptoms, and diagnoses is painstaking and hampers development of software for CDSS. Until easily available and standard sets of terms exist, each development project will need to re-create these lists.

Standards and Methods for Implementation

Standards are an important component of CDSS. As mentioned in the previous section, development of standards for data terminologies and data models is a current field of active research.

Standards. The Logical Observation Identifier Names and Codes[10] is rapidly becoming a standard for the identification of laboratory-test and clinical observations. Systematized Nomenclature of Human Medicine[11] and ICD-9 have been examined for their ability to represent items on the problem list. Health Level Seven is being used successfully to communicate messages, and its Reference Information Model[12] is a robust clinical-data model. The transfer of electronic data between institutions will be enhanced if the data are stored in the Extensible Markup Language[13] format.

Several vendors and research institutions have embraced the Arden Syntax[14] as a means for representing rules for CDSS.

Implementation Issues. As in any setting, CDS implementation in the inpatient setting requires careful attention to several issues. These include technology, training, and knowledge engineering.

Technology Requirements. If the CDSS software is a stand-alone application (for example, access to an information resource such as a dosing adviser) that does not require interfaces to the hospital network, technology issues will be minimal. If, however, the decision-support application is intended to make patient-specific suggestions and interact with a clinician (for example, an application that detects critical laboratory results and notifies the appropriate provider), methods must be provided for the decision-support application to access data from the relevant databases and subsequently to communicate with clinicians. Such interface issues can be extremely complex and often are the major barrier to implementing decision-support applications that truly fit into the clinical workflow. These issues beg an analysis of the computing platform of the decision-support application and the institution's other applications. Such alerting applications must support time triggers (rules that run at certain times), data triggers (rules that run based on new data), or both.

Training and Support Issues. CDSS applications developed for the browser or Windows 95 environments have decreased training issues because the user-interface conventions are standard and thus familiar to most users. Still, CDSS applications can be complex and some level of training and support is likely to be required, especially if the application is key to the clinician's daily work-flow. The issues of training and support for CDSS applications are the same as those for other clinical applications and cannot be overlooked.

Knowledge Engineering. Often, hospitals and other healthcare institutions want to develop decision-support applications for site-specific projects. Besides the technology issues involved in such an effort, gaining and maintaining the requisite knowledge can be difficult. Usually, domain experts (clinicians, high-level administrators) are the repository of the "knowledge." The programming staff has the responsibility of encoding the knowledge. For most nonmedical domains, the programming requirements are created by systems analysts without much specialized training. However, the medical domain is so complex and content rich that the CDSS programming requirements must be created by specialized knowledge engineers. Ideally, knowledge engineers should have a background in medical informatics and have knowledge of computer science, knowledge representation and dictionary issues, the institution's computer-based data, the organizational structure of the institution, and the workflow in the clinical area where the application will be active.

Implementing CDSS software of any kind is time consuming and expensive. Institutions should be well aware of the effort required and the potential hurdles they will have to leap over.

Critical Functionality

We refer to *knowledge-based clinical decision support* as software that, in some way, has knowledge of medicine embedded in it. It supports clinicians' decision making by "thinking like a physician." We will address this topic shortly. In this section, we address software that assists clinicians' decision making without having explicit knowledge of medicine.

Non-Knowledge-Based Clinical Decision Support.   Since the late 1970s, most hospitals have implemented some computing facilities that assist clinicians in carrying out their work. Even without embedded medical knowledge, these applications help clinicians with their decision making and thus provide decision support. An example is an application that gathers periodically obtained laboratory or physiologic data and displays it in a spreadsheet (flow sheet) or in some graphical fashion. Trends, multisystem problems, and even spurious results may become evident to clinicians when data are presented in this manner.

Access to Patient-Independent Data and Information. Several computing technologies allow clinicians to access easily and automatically a wide variety of reference materials. Many institutions have created online versions of their manuals, policies, procedures, and clinical disease-management guidelines. Improved access to these text sources can improve compliance with local standards of care. Also, with the advent of network- and browser-based hospital information systems, workstations can display commercially available CD-ROM-based information sources such as the *PDR*, *Micromedex*, and *Scientific American Medicine*. Finally, clinicians can use Internet technologies to access the wide variety of resources available on the World Wide Web. Although the quality of information on the web needs to be scrutinized, and clinicians may need to be guided to good sites, using the web as a resource is an exciting way for clinicians to fulfill their information needs.

Access to Patient Data. Results-review applications are the most ubiquitous clinical applications in hospitals. To provide the best care, clinicians need easy access to patients' previous test results and other relevant data. If these data are difficult to access, physicians will be "flying blind" as they care for patients. In addition to simply providing the data, results-review applications may embody some amount of medical knowledge by grouping the data in ways that ease comprehension. We describe such formatted reports below.

E-mail. Electronic mail is becoming ubiquitous and is affecting professional and social interactions in many ways. Increasingly, healthcare institutions are providing their workers with e-mail applications. Administrators and clinicians alike use such applications for a variety of purposes. Clinicians can communicate with each other easily in making and responding to informal consultation requests. E-mail is appealing because of its relative ease (compared with dictating a letter or making a phone call) and the fact that it does not interrupt the recipient. The breadth of the e-mail network and the rapidity with which e-mail messages are read determine the value of this technology at any particular site.

Knowledge-Based Clinical Decision Support. Knowledge-based clinical decision support (KBCDS) is software that incorporates medical knowledge so the application can "think" like a clinician. KBCDS has been the object of study for over forty years and has yielded a variety of theoretical and practical results.

Conceptual Model. "Medical knowledge" is the component that differentiates KBCDS from other clinical software. Somehow, this knowledge must be represented in the computer and must be able to assist the clinician with decision making. The key components of a KBCDS application are shown in Figure 1. The first important component of such an application is the triggering event, the action that sets the KBCDS application into motion. The triggering event may be a user-initiated event, a timed event, or a database filing event. We will see many different kinds of triggering events in the sections that follow. The second major component of a knowledge-based application is the knowledge itself. Most KBCDS applications restrict themselves to

Figure 1. Block Diagram of Knowledge-Based Clinical Decision Support

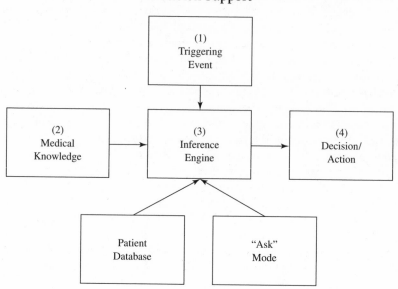

providing decision support for a narrow domain of medicine (critical laboratory-result alerting, blood-gas interpretation, internal-medicine diagnosis). The knowledge in the software can be represented in various ways (as rules, probabilities, neural networks, procedural codes). The third major component of a KBCDS application is the software that actually makes the decision. This component uses the triggering data and the knowledge to "infer" that something is true; thus this piece of software is often called the inference engine. The fourth major component is the decision or action that results from the inference. This decision may be communicated via a page or an e-mail message, or it may be displayed on the computer screen in an interactive application. In some cases, the inference engine may need to access data from the patient database to make its decision, so in these cases the patient database can be considered part of the KBCDS application. If a database is not available, an interactive KBCDS application may have an "ask" mode to acquire additional data from the user.

One class of KBCDS applications signal critical laboratory values. The triggering event would be a new laboratory result, perhaps a serum potassium of 6.5. An example of knowledge in this application would be a rule that states, "Generate an alert if the serum potassium result is greater than 6.0." The inference engine would be able to take the triggering data and infer that an alert is necessary. Some mechanism would be necessary to communicate the alert to the appropriate person. A second example of an alert would be a new hematocrit result of 18 and a rule that states, "Generate an alert if the hematocrit has fallen 10 since the last result." To determine whether the rule is applicable, the inference engine would need to know the patient's previous hematocrit. This information can be obtained from a patient database (or via an "ask" mode). A more subtle trend event would take into account the time between hematocrit determinations and alert if the rate of decline exceeded a certain threshold.[15]

Another class of KBCDS applications is diagnostic programs; here clinicians supply the triggering event (they enter a set of signs or symptoms). The diagnostic knowledge in these applications is represented in a variety of ways (rules,[3] Bayesian statistics,[6] evoking strengths[4]). Most diagnostic programs ask the user for more information rather than query a patient database. The output of such a KBCDS application often is a ranked list of likely diagnoses.

Although conceptually the knowledge base and the inference engine are distinct, they often are tightly coupled. Performance is optimized if two components are coupled but maintenance becomes more difficult.

Categories. Many different kinds of KBCDS applications have been developed over the years to support a wide variety of clinical decision-making situations. These applications can be grouped by the different categories of cases for which a clinician may need help with decision making.[16] Five categories of CDSS applications have been developed; they are described below, and examples of each category are shown in Table 1.

Formatting applications have been designed to help the clinician answer the question, What, in general, is going on with this patient? Several institutions have developed specialized results-review applications to help clinicians care for their hospitalized patients. Although the medical knowledge contained in such programs may not be immediately evident and may be simplistic when compared with the knowledge in other KBCDS applications, the importance of these applications cannot be underestimated. One of a clinician's most important tasks is to review and understand the large amount of data about a patient's physiologic state and therapies. If the data are compiled and presented in a way that facilitates comprehension, the clinician's task is made much easier. In these applications, the medical knowledge is contained in knowing which data to present and in what layout. Examples of such specialized reports include a twenty-four-hour ICU rounds report and a seventy-two-hour summary report in use at LDS Hospital,[17] the "pocket rounds" report in use at Wishard Memorial Hospital,[18] and the sign-out report in use at Brigham and Women's Hospital. Each of these reports may include data from the laboratory, the medications list, intravenous (IV) fluids, intake and outputs, monitors, ventilators, other ICU devices, nurse charting, and radiology. The sign-out program at Brigham and Women's Hospital has been associated with a decrease in adverse events for inpatients who are covered by a physician other than their primary physician.[19]

The question that is asked in *interpreting applications* is, What does this new piece of data mean? Clinicians often interpret new data incorrectly and

Table 1. Examples of Applications of Clinical Decision Support, by Category

Category	Class	Specific Application	Reference
Formatting	Specialized reports	Many, see refs.	17, 18
Interpreting	EKG interpretation	Many, see refs.	21
	Blood-gas interpretation	LDS Hospital	23
	Pulmonary-function-test interpretation	LDS Hospital	17
	Pap-smear interpretation	Autopap	22
	Hemodynamic-data interpretation	LDS Hospital	24
Consulting	Antibiotic selection	Mycin	3
	Internal-medicine diagnosis	Iliad	5
	Internal-medicine diagnosis	Internist-1/QMR	4
	Acute abdominal pain	Dedombal	26, 27
	MI diagnosis	Baxt	29
	Diabetes guideline	Lobach and Hammond	34
	Cholesterol guideline	Tsui et al.	33
	Guidelines for exposure to body fluids	Schriger et al.	35
	ICU mortality risk	APACHE	39
	Chemotherapy	Oncocin	36, 37
	Immunization	Miller et al.	32
Monitoring	Alerting	Kuperman et al.	40
	Alerting	Tate et al.	41
	Alerting	Rind et al.	42
	Alerting	Wagner et al.	43
	Alerting	Shabot et al.	44
	Infectious-disease and antibiotic monitoring	Larsen et al., Evans et al.	45, 46
	Infectious-disease monitoring	Kahn et al.	47
	ADE monitoring	Many	49, 50
	Corollary ordering	Overhage et al.	55
	Monitoring of patients w/ ARDS	Sittig et al.	54
	Utilization review	Nelson and Gardner	51
	Length of stay	Shea et al.	53
Critiquing	Anesthesia	Miller	57
	Ventilator	Miller	56
	Hypertension	Miller and Black	58
	Radiology workup	Harpole et al.	60
	Blood ordering	Gardner et al.	59

several KBCDS applications have been developed to assist with this task. Applications in this category are probably the most developed, and many are in routine clinical use and are available from vendors. High-low flags for laboratory results are the simplest example of this kind of feature. Many of these applications have been developed for ICUs, where the volume of data is larger than in any other hospital setting.[20] Examples in this category are applications that interpret electrocardiograph (EKG) signals,[21] pap smears,[22] pulmonary-function tests,[17] blood-gas results,[23] and hemodynamic data.[24] Many of these applications have been evaluated. For example, some but not all commercial EKG-interpretation programs performed as well as expert cardiologists.[21] In another study, an automatic pap-smear interpretation was superior to methods in current use.[22]

In contrast to interpreting applications, which help a clinician decide what to do about a piece of data, *consulting applications* help the clinician decide what to do about a patient. Consultation applications assist clinicians with diagnosis and treatment; many of these kinds of applications have been built over the years. Examples of applications in this category are diagnostic applications, applications that assist with adherence to treatment guidelines, treatment-plan applications, and applications that attempt to predict patient outcomes.

Diagnostic programs have received much notoriety over the years. As mentioned, Warner's groundbreaking work[1] showed that Bayesian analysis of cardiac-catheterization data was as good as expert cardiologists in the diagnosis of congenital heart disease. Mycin[3] was a program that attempted to diagnose and suggest treatment for meningitis and bacteremia. Mycin pioneered the use of production rules for diagnostic reasoning and spawned a long line of research into diagnostic techniques. Internist-1,[4] which became Quick Medical Reference (QMR),[25] and DXplain[5] used ad hoc knowledge bases to suggest diagnoses. QMR and DXplain persist to this day, but they are used mainly as educational tools. de Dombal[26 27] developed a Bayesian tool to assist with diagnosis of the acute abdomen that was at least as accurate as physicians. Goldman[28] used a simple protocol (derived from a statistical analysis) that was superior to clinicians in the prediction of myocardial infarction (MI), and Baxt[29] developed a neural-network-based program that was also superior to clinicians in the diagnosis of MI.

To date, one difficulty with diagnostic programs is that extra effort is required to invoke their use; they are not part of the clinician's workflow. Ideally, diagnostic applications could be interfaced with electronic medical-record applications to suggest diagnoses that had not yet been considered. However, several difficulties are encountered when trying to interface diagnostic programs and electronic medical-record applications. Also, diagnostic programs still have difficulties. When four computer-based general-medicine diagnostic programs were evaluated,[30] it was found that they made many useful suggestions but they also made many unhelpful suggestions. Such applications may be more distracting than helpful. Finally, much of the data (symptoms, physical findings) that the diagnostic programs need to render their evaluations are not contained in electronic medical-record applications, so redundant entry by clinicians would still be necessary.

Several applications have been developed to help ensure that clinicians treat their patients in accordance with guidelines. Although most of this work applies to the outpatient setting, it is included here for completeness. An overview of the topic has been written by Zielstorff.[31] Examples of applications that have been developed to ensure adherence to guidelines include computer-assisted guidelines for childhood immunization,[32] cholesterol testing,[33] diabetes management,[34] and exposure to body fluids.[35] Many of the programs that provide CDSS for guidelines in the clinical setting have been shown to increase compliance.

Applications that assist with therapy planning have the potential to bring expert care to sites that may not have such expertise. One example, Oncocin,[36 37] suggested chemotherapy treatment (based on protocols) as well as oncologists in a university clinic did. An antibiotic treatment adviser[38] has been developed that reduces costs and length of stay. Therapy-planning programs still are not in widespread use. They would be implemented best as part of order-entry applications.

A final type of consulting application uses statistical models to predict patient outcomes.[39] Such applications could help clinicians decide when to apply scarce resources. Although these models are useful for predicting outcomes for populations of patients, they are not accurate enough to help with critical decisions about individual patients.

Monitoring applications are part of clinical-information systems. They examine all new data and use a rule base to identify important clinical events. Thus, they assure that clinicians do not overlook any important data.

There are several examples of monitoring applications. Alerting applications detect critical laboratory results and automatically notify the patient's provider.[40 41 42 43 44] Critical-alert conditions are associated with significantly higher ICU and hospital mortality and longer ICU stays.[44] Alerting applications have been shown to reduce delays in treating patients and to increase the frequency with which patients are treated appropriately.

Monitoring applications related to infectious disease identify patients who (1) have a reportable disease, (2) are not receiving appropriate antibiotics (based on cost or cultural sensitivities or both), (3) are receiving antibiotics for too long, (4) have hospital-acquired infections, and (5) should have antibiotics prior to surgery.[45 46 47] Monitoring applications are also used to detect potential problems in respiratory therapy,[48] to detect potential adverse drug events (ADEs),[49 50] to screen for inappropriate inpatient utilization,[51] to identify patients who may have tuberculosis but are not in isolation rooms,[52] to inform clinicians of the expected length of stay,[53] and to review the status of and suggest treatment for patients with adult respiratory-distress syndrome (ARDS).[54] Additionally, there are several monitoring features in physician order-entry applications. Examples are features that require orders to be complete and features that suggest orders in light of other orders.[55]

Critiquing applications review proposed therapies or diagnostic studies and offer a comment to the clinician. Miller has developed critiquing applications for ventilatory management,[56] anesthesia management,[57] and hypertension treatment,[58] but these programs have never been put into routine clinical use. Gardner[59] developed a blood-ordering critiquing application, and Harpole[60] evaluated a radiology-ordering critiquing application; both of these are in clinical use.

Impact of Decision Support in Hospital and Critical Care Settings

The impact of CDS applications can be measured in several ways. At a minimum, CDSS applications should generate accurate decisions. For example, diagnostic programs should generate appropriate diagnoses; alerting applications should generate alerts correctly, and critiquing applications should generate a critique in the same way as an expert consultant would. Many of the references at the end of this article are evaluations of the correctness (as well as descriptions) of CDSS applications.

For CDSS applications in clinical use, other evaluation measures can be applied. One measure of impact is use: how many alerts were generated,[48] how many interpretations were generated,[20] how often was a guideline program accessed. A second evaluation measure is the impact on the process of medical care. Examples of CDSS applications that have changed the process of medical care are those that improve compliance with care guidelines[34] and those that increase the appropriateness of therapy.[41]

The most important kind of evaluation study is one that measures impact on patient outcomes—either the cost or the quality of medical care. CDSS applications that have had a measurable impact on patient outcomes include an alerting application that was associated with better renal function at discharge[42] and an antibiotic adviser that decreased cost and length of stay.[38] Many methodological difficulties are encountered in performing sound evaluations of CDSS applications. Hunt and colleagues[61] reviewed the literature on the effect of CDSS applications on physician performance and patient outcomes. Only sixty-eight articles (forty since 1992) met their strict criteria for methodological soundness. Many of the articles involved dosing assistance and many involved reminders for preventive care (largely in the outpatient setting). Only fourteen of the sixty-eight assessed patient outcomes, and only six were found to have a benefit. Although a lot of benefit can be documented in the absence of rigorous studies, much work needs to be done to demonstrate the positive impact of CDSS applications. CDSS applications should be evaluated as would any other medical technology.

Future Trends for Clinical Decision Support in the Inpatient Setting

Over the next decade, managed care and the need for improved and consistent clinical decision making will promote the movement of CDSS applications from the research and "proof-of-concept" stage into wider practice. However, several "enabling technologies" will similarly need to advance. For example, electronic medical records (EMRs) are an important application that enables much of the benefit of CDSS to be realized. If EMRs become widespread, many more CDSS can be expected too. Similarly, work on standards and interfaces will need to advance if the benefits of CDSS are to be realized.

The delivery of alerts and reminders to caregivers is an area where progress is being made. Methods used in the past include flashing lights on nursing units, terminal messages, and e-mail. Newer applications can deliver automated alert, advisory, and critiquing messages directly to clinicians' pagers and pocket computers over a wireless network.[62] These applications now allow caregivers to respond to messages using a reliable two-way wireless medium. Other research is examining the most appropriate way to deliver any particular message. Some applications allow users to "subscribe" to certain alerts and decide the manner in which they wish to be notified (for example, e-mail or page).

To reap all the benefits of CDSS, the manner in which guidelines are represented in the computer[31] and interact with an EMR will need further research. Research will continue in knowledge representation, and more complex medical decision making (diagnosis, prediction rules) will become possible with neural networks and advanced statistical techniques.

Access to data will become easier (for example, via the Internet), and standard technologies will permit different data types to be integrated more easily (for example, viewing images on a browser). These advances in technologies will offer a myriad of opportunities.

In general, decision-support tools will move out of the research and development environment and become part of a "cockpit" for clinicians as they try to deliver the highest quality, most efficient care.

References

1. Warner, H. R., Jr. "A Mathematical Approach to Medical Diagnosis: Application to Congenital Heart Disease." *Journal of the American Medical Association,* 1961, *177* (3), 75–81.
2. Ledley, R. S., and Lusted, L. B. "Reasoning Foundations of Medical Diagnosis." *Science,* 1959, *130,* 9–21. (Reprinted in *MD Computing,* 1991, *8* (5), 300–315.)
3. Shortliffe, E. H., Davis, R., Axline, S. G., Buchanan, B. G., Green, C. C., Cohen, S. N. "Computer-Based Consultations in Clinical Therapeutics: Explanation and Rule Acquisition Capabilities of the MYCIN System." *Computers and Biomedical Research,* 1975, *8* (4), 303–320.
4. Miller, R. A., Pople, H. E., Jr., and Myers, J. D. "Internist-1, an Experimental Computer-Based Diagnostic Consultant for General Internal Medicine." *New England Journal of Medicine,* 1982, *307* (8), 468–476.

5. Barnett, G. O., Cimino, J. J., Hupp, J. A., and Hoffer, E. P. "DXplain: An Evolving Diagnostic Decision-Support System." *Journal of the American Medical Association,* 1987, *258* (1), 67–74.
6. Warner, H. R., Jr. "Iliad: Moving Medical Decision-Making into New Frontiers." *Methods of Information in Medicine,* 1989, *28* (4), 370–372.
7. Reisman, Y. "Computer Based Clinical Decision Aids: A Review of Methods and Assessment of Systems." *Medical Informatics,* 1996, *21* (3), 179–197.
8. Kassirer, J. P. "Diagnostic Reasoning." *Annals of Internal Medicine,* 1989, *110* (11), 893–900.
9. Hripcsak, G., Kuperman, G. J., and Friedman, C. "Extracting Findings from Narrative Reports: Software Transferability and Sources of Physician Disagreement." *Methods of Information in Medicine,* 1998, *37* (1), 1–7.
10. Huff, S. M., and others. "Development of the Logical Observation Identifier Names and Codes (LOINC) Vocabulary." *Journal of the American Medical Informatics Association,* 5 (3), 276–292.
11. Lussier, Y. A., Rothwell, D. J., and Cote, R. A. "The SNOMED Model: A Knowledge Source for the Controlled Terminology of the Computerized Patient Record." *Methods of Information in Medicine,* 1998, *37* (2), 161–164.
12. Jenders, R. A., Sujansky, W., Broverman, C. A., and Chadwick, M. "Towards Improved Knowledge Sharing: Assessment of the HL7 Reference Information Model to Support Medical Logic Module Queries." *Proceedings of the AMIA Annual Fall Symposium,* 1997, 308–312.
13. Dudeck, J. "Aspects of Implementing and Harmonizing Healthcare Communication Standards." *International Journal of Medical Informatics,* 1998, *48* (1–3), 163–171.
14. Hripcsak, G., Ludemann, P., Pryor, T. A., Wigertz, O. B., and Clayton, P. D. "Rationale for the Arden Syntax." *Computers and Biomedical Research,* 1994, *27* (4), 291–324.
15. Shabot, M. M., LoBue, M., Leyerle, B. J, and Dubin, S. B. "Inferencing Strategies for Automated Alerts on Critically Abnormal Laboratory and Blood Gas Data." *Proceedings of the Annual Symposium on Computer Applications in Medical Care,* 1989, *13,* 54–57.
16. http://www.informatics-review.com/thoughts/interactions.html
17. Kuperman, G. J., Gardner, R. M., and Pryor, T. A. *HELP: A Dynamic Hospital Information System.* New York: Springer-Verlag, 1991.
18. McDonald, C. J., Tierney, W. M., Martin, D. K., and Overhage, J. M. "The Regenstrief Medical Record System: 20 Years of Experience in Hospitals, Clinics and Neighborhood Health Centers." *MD Computing,* 1992, *9* (4), 206–217.
19. Petersen, L. A., Orav, E. J., Teich, J. M., O'Neil, A. C., and Brennan, T. A. "Using a Computerized Sign-Out Program to Improve Continuity of Inpatient Care and Prevent Adverse Events." *Joint Commission Journal on Quality Improvement,* 1998, *24* (2), 77–87.
20. Clemmer, T. P., and Gardner, R. M. "Data Gathering, Analysis, and Display in Critical Care Medicine." *Respiratory Care,* 1985, *30,* 586–598.
21. Willems, J. L., and others. "The Diagnostic Performance of Computer Programs for the Interpretation of Electrocardiograms." *New England Journal of Medicine,* 1991, *325* (25), 1767–1773.
22. Wilbur, D. C., Prey, M. U., Miller, W. M., Pawlick, G. F., and Colgan, T. J. "The AutoPap System for Primary Screening in Cervical Cytology. Comparing the Results of a Prospective, Intended-Use Study with Routine Manual Practice." *Acta Cytologica,* 1998, *42* (1), 214–220.
23. Gardner, R. M., Cannon, G. H., Morris, A. H., Olsen, K. R., and Price, G. A. "Computerized Blood Gas Interpretation and Reporting System." *IEEE Computing,* 1975, *8* (1), 39–45.
24. Gardner, R. M. "Computerized Management of Intensive Care Patients." *MD Computing,* 1986, *3* (1), 36–51.
25. Bankowitz, R. A., McNeil, M. A., Challinor, S. M., Parker, R. C., Kapoor, W. N., and Miller, R. A. "A Computer-Assisted Medical Diagnostic Consultation Service: Implementation and Prospective Evaluation of a Prototype. *Annals of Internal Medicine,* 1989, *110* (10), 824–832.

26. de Dombal, F. T., Horrocks, J. C., Staniland, J. R., and Guillou, P. J. "Construction and Uses of an E-Database of Clinical Information Concerning 600 Patients with Acute Abdominal Pain." *Proceedings of the Royal Society of Medicine,* 1971, *64* (9), 978.

27. deDombal, F. T., Leaper, D. J., Staniland, J. R., McCann, A. P., and Horrocks, J. C. "Computer-Aided Diagnosis of Acute Abdominal Pain." *British Medical Journal,* 1972, *2* (5804), 9–13.

28. Goldman, L., and others. "A Computer Protocol to Predict Myocardial Infarction in Emergency Department Patients with Chest Pain." *New England Journal of Medicine,* 1988, *318* (13), 797–803.

29. Baxt, W. G. "Use of an Artificial Neural Network for the Diagnosis of Myocardial Infarction." *Annals of Internal Medicine,* 1991, *115* (11), 843–848.

30. Berner, E. S., and others. "Performance of Four Computer-Based Diagnostic Systems." *New England Journal of Medicine,* 1994, *330* (25), 1792–1796.

31. Zielstorff, R. D. "Online Practice Guidelines: Issues, Obstacles, and Future Prospects." *Journal of the American Medical Informatics Association,* 1998, *5* (3), 227–236.

32. Miller, P. L., Frawley, S. J., Sayward, F. G., Yasnoff, W. A., Duncan, L., and Fleming, D. W. "Combining Tabular, Rule-Based, and Procedural Knowledge in Computer-Based Guidelines for Childhood Immunization." *Computer Biomedical Research,* 1997, *30* (3), 211–231.

33. Tsui, F. C., Wagner, M. M., and Thompson, M. E. "Implementing NCEP Guidelines in a Web-Based Disease-Management System." *Proceedings of the AMIA Annual Fall Symposium,* 1997, 764–768.

34. Lobach, D. F., and Hammond, W. E. "Computerized Decision Support Based on a Clinical Practice Guideline Improves Compliance with Care Standards." *American Journal of Medicine,* 1997, *102* (1), 89–98.

35. Schriger, D. L., Baraff, L. J., Rogers, W. H., and Cretin, S. "Implementation of Clinical Guidelines Using a Computer Charting System: Effect on the Initial Care of Health Care Workers Exposed to Body Fluids." *Journal of the American Medical Society,* 1997, *278* (19), 1585–1590.

36. Hickam, D. H., Shortliffe, E. H., Bischoff, M. B., Scott, A. C., and Jacobs, C. D. "The Treatment Advice of a Computer-Based Cancer Chemotherapy Protocol Advisor." *Annals of Internal Medicine,* 1985, *103* (6, pt. 1), 928–936.

37. Langlotz, C. P., Fagan, L. M., Tu, S. W., Sikic, B. I., and Shortliffe, E. H. "A Therapy Planning Architecture That Combines Decision Theory and Artificial Intelligence Techniques." *Computer Biomedical Research,* 1987, *20* (3), 279–303.

38. Evans, R. S., Pestotnik, S. L., Classen, D. C., Clemmer, T. P., Weaver, L. K., Orme, J. F., Jr., Lloyd, J. F., and Burke, J. P. "A Computer-Assisted Management Program for Antibiotics and Other Antiinfective Agents." *New England Journal of Medicine,* 1998, *338* (4), 232–238.

39. Zimmerman, J. E., Wagner, D. P., Draper, E. A., Wright, L., Alzola, C., and Knaus, W. A. "Evaluation of Acute Physiology and Chronic Health Evaluation III Predictions of Hospital Mortality in an Independent Database." *Critical Care Medicine,* 1998, *26* (8), 1317–1326.

40. Kuperman, G. J., Teich, J. M., Bates, D. W., Hiltz, F. L., Hurley, J. M., Lee, R. Y., and Paterno, M. D. "Detecting Alerts, Notifying the Physician, and Offering Action Items: A Comprehensive Alerting System." *Proceedings of the AMIA Annual Fall Symposium,* 1996, 704–708.

41. Tate, K. E., Gardner, R. M., and Weaver, L. K. "A Computerized Laboratory Alerting System." *MD Computing,* 1990, *7* (5), 296–301.

42. Rind, D. M., Safran, C., Phillips, R. S., Wang, Q., Calkins, D. R., Delbanco, T. L., Bleich, H. L., and Slack, W. V. "Effect of Computer-Based Alerts on the Treatment and Outcomes of Hospitalized Patients." *Archives of Internal Medicine,* 1994, *154* (13), 1511–1517.

43. Wagner, M. M., Pankaskie, M., Hogan, W., Tsui, F. C., Eisenstadt, S. A., Rodriguez, E., and Vries, J. K. "Clinical Event Monitoring at the University of Pittsburgh." *Proceedings of the AMIA Annual Fall Symposium,* 1997, 188–192.

44. Shabot, M. M., LoBue, M., Leyerle, B. J., and Dubin, S. B. "Decision Support Alerts for Clinical Laboratory and Blood Gas Data." *International Journal of Clinical Monitoring and Computing,* 1990, 7 (1), 27–31.

45. Larsen, R. A., Evans, R. S., Burke, J. P., Pestotnik, S. L., Gardner, R. M., and Classen, D. C. "Improved Perioperative Antibiotic Use and Reduced Surgical Wound Infections Through Use of Computer Decision Analysis." 1989, *10* (7), 316–320.

46. Evans, R. S., and others. "Computer Surveillance of Hospital-Acquired Infections and Antibiotic Use." *Journal of the American Medical Association,* 1986, *256* (8), 1007–1011.

47. Kahn, M. G., Steib, S. A., Fraser, V. J., and Dunagan, W. C. "An Expert System for Culture-Based Infection Control Surveillance." *Proceedings of the Annual Symposium on Computer Applications in Medical Care,* 1993, 171–175.

48. Elliot, C. G. "Computer-Assisted Quality Assurance: Development and Performance of a Respiratory Care Program." *QRB Quality Review Bulletin,* 1991, *17,* 85–90.

49. Evans, R. S., Pestotnik, S. L., Classen, D. C., Bass, S. B., Menlove, R. L., Gardner, R. M., and Burke, J. P. "Development of a Computerized Adverse Drug Event Monitor." *Proceedings of the Annual Symposium on Computer Applications in Medical Care,* 1991, 23–27.

50. Jha, A. K., and others. "Identifying Adverse Drug Events: Development of a Computer-Based Monitor and Comparison with Chart Review and Stimulated Voluntary Report." *Journal of the American Medical Informatics Association,* 1998, *5* (3), 305–314.

51. Nelson, B. D., and Gardner, R. M. "Decision Support for Concurrent Utilization Review Using a Help-Embedded Expert System." *Proceedings of the Annual Symposium on Computer Applications in Medical Care,* 1993, 176–182.

52. Knirsch, C. A., Jain, N. L., Pablos-Mendez, A., Friedman, C., and Hripcsak, G. "Respiratory Isolation of Tuberculosis Patients Using Clinical Guidelines and an Automated Clinical Decision Support System." *Infection Control and Hospital Epidemiology,* 1998, *19* (2), 94–100.

53. Shea, S., Sideli, R. V., DuMouchel, W., Pulver, G., Arons, R. R., and Clayton, P. D. "Computer-Generated Informational Messages Directed to Physicians: Effect on Length of Hospital Stay." *Journal of the American Medical Informatics Association,* 1995, *2* (1), 58–64.

54. Sittig, D. F., Pace, N. L., Gardner, R. M., Beck, E., and Morris, A. H. "Implementation of a Computerized Patient Advice System Using the HELP Clinical Information System." *Computer Biomedical Research,* 1989, 22 (5), 474–487.

55. Overhage, J. M., Tierney, W. M., Zhou, X. H., and McDonald, C. J. "A Randomized Trial of 'Corollary Orders' to Prevent Errors of Omission." *Journal of the American Medical Informatics Association,* 1997, *4* (5), 364–375.

56. Miller, P. L. "Extending Computer-Based Critiquing to a New Domain: ATTENDING, ESSENTIAL-ATTENDING, and VQ-ATTENDING." *International Journal of Clinical Monitoring and Computing,* 1986, *2* (3), 135–142.

57. Miller, P. L. "Critiquing Anesthetic Management: The 'ATTENDING' Computer System." *Anesthesiology,* 1983, *58,* 362–369.

58. Miller, P. L., and Black, H. R. "HT-ATTENDING. Critiquing the Pharmacologic Management of Essential Hypertension." *Journal of Medical Systems,* 1984, 8 (3), 181–187.

59. Gardner, R. M., Golubjatnikov, O. K., Laub, R. M., Jacobson, J. T., and Evans, R. S. "Computer-Critiqued Blood Ordering Using the HELP System." *Computer Biomedical Research,* 1990, 23 (6), 514–528.

60. Harpole, L. H., Khorasani, R., Fiskio, J., Kuperman, G. J., and Bates, D. W. "Automated Evidence-Based Critiquing of Orders for Abdominal Radiographs: Impact on Utilization and Appropriateness." *Journal of the American Medical Informatics Association,* 1997, *4* (6), 511–521.

61. Hunt, D. L., Haynes, R. B., Hanna, S. E., and Smith, K. "Effects of Computer-Based Clinical Decision Support Systems on Physician Performance and Patient Outcomes: A Systematic Review." *Journal of the American Medical Association,* 1998, *280* (15), 1339–1346.

62. Shabot, M. M., and LoBue, M. "Real-Time Wireless Decision Support Alerts on a Palmtop PDA." *Proceedings of the Annual Symposium on Computer Applications in Medical Care,* 1995, *19,* 174–177.

About the Authors

Gilad J. Kuperman, M.D., Ph.D., is clinical systems designer for Partners Healthcare System, Chestnut Hill, MA.

Dean F. Sittig, Ph.D., is the corporate manager of clinical systems research and development at Partners Healthcare System, Chestnut Hill, Massachusetts.

M. Michael Shabot, M.D., FACS, FCCM, FACMI, is the medical director for enterprise information services and director of surgical intensive care at Cedars-Sinai Medical Center, Los Angeles.

Inpatient Order Management

Jonathan M. Teich, M.D., Ph.D.

Inpatient provider order entry (POE) is one of the most effective tools for the implementation of powerful clinical decision support. In POE, doctors and other clinical providers enter all orders directly into the computer. Although the implementation of order entry is complex and perilous, the potential benefits for patient care and cost reduction can be tremendous. This chapter reviews some of the considerations in the design and implementation of POE, and examines some of the ways that clinical decision support is introduced into a POE system.

An Example

To set the stage for this article and to give a general sense of how inpatient order entry uses decision support, let us start with an example. Consider the physician who writes a new order for digoxin to be given to her patient. The physician goes to the computer workstation, selects medication orders, and chooses digoxin. Immediately, the computer, acting on preprogrammed rules, performs a series of tests to see whether these new data have any important consequences. The computer checks for allergies to digoxin and related drugs, looks for interactions between digoxin and any of the patient's other medications, ensures that this order does not duplicate another medication order, checks relevant laboratory tests to see whether they portend any hazard if digoxin is administered, and checks for any clinical rules designed to steer the physician to a different drug.

Suppose this patient's current potassium level is 3.2. This is not such a drastically low level that it would prompt immediate alarm in the laboratory, but patients taking digoxin are especially sensitive to even moderate hypokalemia. The computer's clinical decision support system notes the worrisome result and generates an intervention. The computer displays a screen indicating the concern, shows the relevant laboratory-test result, and offers a choice of reasonable alternatives—in this case, canceling the digoxin order, ordering more potassium, ordering a new potassium test, or proceeding without any change.

The doctor considers the suggestions, decides to order more potassium, and then continues with the digoxin order. Before the order is completed, the computer helps in several other ways. It offers a recommended dose and frequency for the digoxin order, adjusted for the patient's renal status. Relevant laboratory results are displayed right on the ordering screen. At the end of the order, if any additional orders are called for as a consequence of this order (such as drug-level monitoring),[1] a pop-up screen will ask the doctor whether she wishes to add those consequent orders.

The Computer-Human Partnership

In the example above, hypokalemia and renal failure are concepts that the doctor understands very well. The computer's important contribution is reminding the doctor, at exactly the time of ordering, that these conditions exist in this particular patient. For a doctor who takes care of many patients concurrently, dealing with hundreds or thousands of data items for each one, the problem is not so much not knowing what to do with information. Rather, it is filtering all the data efficiently enough to know that important information is present at all.

This relationship between data and knowledge is the essence of the ideal partnership between computers and humans. Physicians are better at making diagnoses and understanding the processes of care. Computers are much better at storing and remembering large numbers of facts and screening each one on the basis of preprogrammed rules. The computer can distill the most important facts to bring to the physician's attention. In this role, the computer is not so much an expert consultant, possessing superior clinical knowledge. Rather, the computer is more like a highly attentive medical student—not able to deal independently with every aspect of the patient's care, but meticulous enough to keep track of all the patient's data and skilled enough to know when something is important enough to bring to the physician's attention. This advanced communication function is the basis of much of the successful impact of clinical decision support in POE.

Using POE, the computer can assist in these ways:

- Preventing adverse events through order checking and presenting reminders such as those described above
- Promoting optimal care through the use of order sets, templates, and disease-management algorithms
- Promoting cost-effective care by sensing excess use and suggesting alternatives
- Providing proactive workup guidance, through disease-management algorithms

Historical Perspective

The role of order entry in a medical information-management system was recognized very early. In 1970, Collen listed it as one of the key components of a clinical-information system and also recommended that orders be entered directly by physicians.[2] Implementation of successful POE systems, however, has been slow and incomplete.

One of the earliest commercial systems was developed by Technicon (commonly called TDS, and currently owned by Eclipsys Corp.). TDS is still the most frequently used POE vendor, although only a handful of its sites are using POE. The literature contains many references to unsuccessful implementations of POE systems from a variety of vendors,[3 4 5] although some of these succeeded on the second try. For the most part, the original systems failed because the design did not fit the physicians' practice patterns or because leadership backing for the project was uncertain (or both).

Academic medical informatics departments have been responsible for much of the advancement of clinical decision support in POE.[6] Ordering systems first arose at two of the oldest and most respected academic medical informatics sites: the Regenstrief Institute in Indiana and LDS Hospital in Utah. The Indiana team in particular has published extensively on the effectiveness of their rule-based system in guiding physicians' orders[7] and in reducing inpatient charges.[8] The Utah group developed order entry specifically for blood products[9] and showed that the correct use of these products increased dramatically as a result. In the 1990s, Brigham and Women's Hospital in Boston developed a comprehensive POE system[10] and demonstrated, in a series of articles, that its decision-support features reduced medication costs[10] and significantly reduced adverse drug events.[12] More recently, Vanderbilt University developed a POE system with new decision-support features.[13]

Perhaps prompted by these study results, an increasing number of vendors are now starting to offer ordering systems as part of their product line. Nonetheless, POE is still the exception rather than the rule, even in hospitals that employ comprehensive electronic medical records. A survey[14] indicated that although 32 percent of the hospitals studied stated they had at least some POE, only one-fifth of these hospitals (22 out of 365, or 6 percent of the overall survey group) had as many as half their physicians using it.

Why Order Entry?

A hospital may wish to implement POE for many reasons before it even thinks about clinical decision support. Orders typed on the computer are more legible than those written by hand, which improves speed and convenience of handling and prevents transcription errors. Orders entered into a computer system can be routed in various directions immediately. A medication order written by a physician by hand may go to the unit secretary first, then to the nurse, then finally to the pharmacy, at which time the pharmacist can begin to prepare the medication. An order entered directly into the computer can go simultaneously to the nurse, the unit secretary, and the pharmacist, and perhaps even conveyed directly to the pharmacy information system; the medication can be ready by the time the nurse has read the order.

POE adds considerable convenience and efficiency in hospitals where one doctor may have patients on several floors. Orders can be entered from any workstation in the hospital; the doctor does not need to go to a patient's unit and find the chart before she can write orders (especially important if the patient and the chart are currently off the unit). Because of this remote-access capability, physicians have less need to give verbal orders or telephone orders to the nurse, thus eliminating a source of communications breakdown and transcription error.

Clinical decision support can have such a large impact that it has become a compelling reason, all by itself, for a hospital to consider the implementation of POE. This high impact is related to the way patient care is directed in a hospital. Practically, an inpatient physician affects his patient in one of three ways. He can perform a procedure or an operation on the patient; he can communicate with, listen to, and educate the patient; or he can write orders for medications, tests, and other therapies. In many cases, orders are the primary means of directing therapy for the patient. Because the computer is "in series" with the physician, critiquing and assisting orders before they ever affect the patient, potential errors and adverse events are prevented in a timely fashion.

Why Not Order Entry?

If all the above advantages were available at no cost and with no pain, many more hospitals would immediately implement a POE system. However, this is not the case. Order entry is a major change in the way doctors and institutions do their work. Sufficient workstations must be deployed so that doctors and nurses can conveniently find a place to enter orders whenever necessary. Finding time to train busy physicians to enter data on the computer can be difficult. Even with training, implementation of POE changes patterns that the doctor may have built up over many years. Resistance to such workflow change is natural, so compelling advantages have to be demonstrated. Finally, if the system slows down the ordering process or takes up too much of the doctor's time, it is likely to be rejected out of hand.

For this reason, order entry is not a project undertaken lightly. Careful attention must be given to system design, preimplementation groundwork, training, and postimplementation support.

Critical Design Requirements

Several issues impact upon the design and implementation of successful POE systems. Most important among these are end-user issues including comprehensiveness, ease of use, and added value for the end user. I will discuss each of these in turn.

Comprehensiveness. "Straddle" between computerized and handwritten orders can cause problems. It is inconvenient to have to write some types of orders on paper, while other orders are entered into the computer. It also can cause confusion—should this order go on paper or in the computer?—which can nullify many of the advantages of POE. Although some benefits can still be obtained by an ordering system devoted to a single area, such as radiology, greater benefits accrue when the computer is used for all orders. Another kind of straddle can occur in the implementation period; some patients in a unit may be on computerized orders while others are on handwritten orders. Through rapid rollout and appropriate segmentation, a hospital should eliminate straddle as rapidly as possible.

Ease of Use and Speed of Operation. Ease of use and speed of operation go hand in hand. The computer system should make it as easy as possible to enter orders. By processing input quickly and by providing friendly, intuitive screen navigation, the computer can make it nearly as easy to use POE as it is to scribble an order down on a sheet of paper. By providing on-screen "quick choices" for the most common orders and parameters, and templates to guide physicians through commonly used collections of orders, the POE system can in many cases be easier than handwriting.[8] The same factors enhance the speed of the system's operation. At the outset of a POE implementation, order entry will normally be significantly slower than handwriting.[13] It is critical to get over the learning curve quickly in order to restore or enhance the physician's most precious commodity, time.

At the same time that the system is trying to make common ordering as easy and as fast as possible, it must also permit any reasonable order to be entered, even if it involves unusual values for complex parameters. These two requirements can be in conflict, and careful system design is required to balance them.

In a system this complex, it is also important that the physician be comfortable with the program's operation. The physician must be able to be absolutely clear about whether a given order has been completely entered, whether it represents exactly what the physician had in mind, which orders have not been signed, which orders are waiting for cosign or renewal, and so on. The same is true for the nurse who receives and executes the orders. Because the nurse will normally receive the orders through the computer, he must be able to easily and clearly understand which orders have and which have not yet been processed.

Added Value. Many helpful pieces of information can be presented on the ordering screen to make the physician's life easier. A display of relevant laboratory values provides important information to guide the current order without making the physician go to a different application to look for it. The same is true for displays of other patient data, such as drug allergies and current active medications. Buttons on the screen can be made to access reference information about drugs and tests, hospital policies, and comprehensive cost information. And, of course, POE interventions that prevent errors are a major source of added value. A physician who orders a drug to which the patient is allergic will appreciate having the fact pointed out quietly by the computer before an untoward event occurs.

Design Features

Several components are crucial in any decision-support intervention for POE. These include three functional steps (triggering, presentation, and action items) and three sources of data (knowledge base, order profile, and clinical database).

Triggering. The computer executes logic after certain trigger transactions; the logic then checks the current process and determines whether it needs to interrupt the process with an intervention screen. This logic should run as soon as it has enough information to do so. Some interventions can be triggered as soon as the major item (medication name, test name, blood product) has been identified: for example, a drug-allergy warning should be presented as soon as the name of the medication is known. Other interventions need to wait until certain parameters (dose, frequency, test time, reasons) have been entered. Still others (new items to cosign, for example) are best triggered at the start of an entire order session or even asynchronously by alerting the physician when a newly filed laboratory result requires a change in orders.[15]

Presentation. If the logic determines that an intervention screen or alert is necessary, the screen should include (1) the order, partial order, or process that has caused the concern, (2) a description of the warning, (3) any other relevant data that were used by the logic, (4) a link to a deeper explanation of the intervention if necessary, and (5) a list of remedial actions that the user can select. See Figure 1. It is also useful to include the rule's "owner"—the clinical leader or group that has deemed the intervention necessary—in case the ordering provider has questions about the intervention (see the discussion of rules governance below).

Action Items. When the computer presents an intervention, it can suggest various actions that the physician can take to deal with the situation. These actions typically are to modify or cancel the current order, to modify or cancel a previously entered order, or to create a new order. In most cases, the doctor should be allowed to override any computer recommendation. In more serious cases, such as chemotherapy-dose warnings, another physician must verify an override.[16] When the doctor creates the new or modified order, the computer must check that order as well. For example, if a new drug is chosen as a result of a substitute-therapy intervention, the new drug must be checked for allergies and interactions.

Knowledge Base. The knowledge base stores the rules and logic that describe when interventions will occur and how they will be presented. An efficient knowledge base allows interventions to be added, modified, and deleted easily, as clinical conditions change. Rather than "hard coding" specific interventions, they should be written so that data tables and struc-

Figure 1. A Typical Intervention Screen

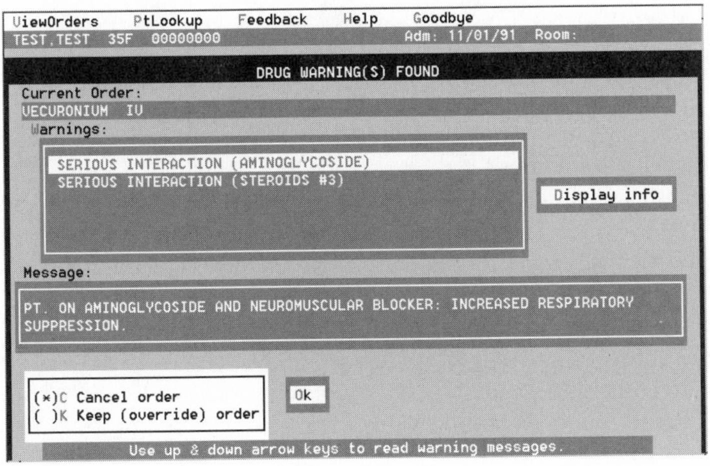

```
 ViewOrders   PtLookup   Feedback   Help    Goodbye
 TEST.TEST  35F  00000000                 Adm: 11/01/91  Room:
                        DRUG WARNING(S) FOUND
 Current Order:
 VECURONIUM   IV
   Warnings:
    ┌─────────────────────────────────────────────────┐
    │ SERIOUS INTERACTION (AMINOGLYCOSIDE)             │
    │ SERIOUS INTERACTION (STEROIDS #3)                │      ┌──────────────┐
    │                                                  │      │ Display info │
    │                                                  │      └──────────────┘
    └─────────────────────────────────────────────────┘
 Message:
    ┌─────────────────────────────────────────────────────────────────┐
    │ PT. ON AMINOGLYCOSIDE AND NEUROMUSCULAR BLOCKER: INCREASED RESPIRATORY │
    │ SUPPRESSION.                                                      │
    └─────────────────────────────────────────────────────────────────┘

    ┌────────────────────────┐   ┌────┐
    │ (×)C Cancel order      │   │ Ok │
    │ ( )K Keep (override) order │ └────┘
    └────────────────────────┘
          Use up & down arrow keys to read warning messages.
```

tures containing the knowledge requirements of specific situations are used. An analyst can make new rules by modifying the tables instead of the computer's code.

Order Profiles. The order profile is the set of all active orders in a given context. Order entry is complicated by the fact that an inpatient may have one profile of current active orders, another profile that will become active after an impending transfer or surgical procedure, and still another that applies when the patient is out of the hospital. A new order may apply to any one of these or to several profiles simultaneously. Intervention logic must carefully determine which profile is applicable, especially when checking the interactions of two orders.

Clinical Database. Decision-support logic compares an order or profile to other relevant data. As more types of data become available in coded form, more sophisticated interventions become possible. For example, a diagnosis-specific order set can be triggered from a coded diagnosis entered on admission; anticoagulation reminders can be based on knowledge that the patient had an orthopedic surgical procedure; a fever workup or suggested antibiotic change can be facilitated when an elevated temperature is entered. Laboratory results, current length of stay, coded historical-problem lists, x-ray and diagnostic-study results have all been used to improve the sensitivity and specificity of interventions in POE.

Another source of important additional data is the medication administration record (MAR), used by nurses to document when drugs are given or held. When an order calls for a medication to be given on an as-needed basis, an electronic MAR provides important information about the actual dosing. This is an important source of data for identifying and preventing potential overdoses and drug interactions.

Classes of Decision Support

Because so much of a patient's care plan is expressed through orders, many interventions can be brought into the ordering process. My colleagues and I have previously published a breakdown of decision-support interventions by categories;[17] the categories relevant to POE are presented here. Major categories of interventions can be identified by using that outline. Almost all have been implemented in at least some of the major academic or commercial systems.[18 6 8 12 19 20] The category breakdown has implications for persons designing or reviewing POE systems: the triggering, presentation, and action items are similar for interventions in the same category.

Substitute-therapy checks include direct one-for-one alternatives, such as recommending a less costly drug in place of the drug that has been entered. This intervention is triggered when a major item is selected; the recommended action changes the current order's major item (medication or test) or parameters (dose or time).

Structured ordering (with feedback) uses a structured form to obtain additional information about the current action, such as the reasons for ordering a diagnostic study or a blood product. The computer then assesses the correctness of that action in that setting. This intervention is effective for restricting the use of expensive antibiotics to critical situations or for ensuring that radiology tests are used for appropriate reasons.[21 22]

Drug-family processing requires that orderable drugs be grouped into families, which have a common property; they may be cross-allergenic, have the same drug interactions, or be in a common therapeutic class. When a medication is selected as a major item, the computer can rapidly check to see whether the relevant families are already "primed" (for example, whether an allergy to medications in that family has previously been entered) and can present an intervention screen if necessary. Drug-family tables facilitate rule maintenance as new drugs are released. A number of commercial vendors offer databases that include drug-family groupings.

Parameter checking ensures correctness of specific order parameters such as doses, ventilator settings, and test times. Triggering usually occurs when the parameter is entered or when the order is completed. In some cases, logic runs when the major item is identified, and the presentation is integral to the ordering screen in the form of recommended dose lists or ventilator settings. Having logic run when the major item is identified is especially useful in guiding medication ordering for patients with renal failure.[11]

Excessive-utilization checks reveal when laboratory or diagnostic tests are ordered too frequently or when the cumulative dosage of an ordered medication or ingredient is excessive. In the outpatient arena, this feature can be used to check costs accumulated against a payer's maximum benefit.

Relevant-information displays are triggered when the major item is identified. These interventions present the information, such as relevant laboratory results, allergies, or reference information, directly on the ordering screen.

Time-based checking is the primary means of detecting errors of omission. It can be used to alert the physician when orders will expire if not renewed, when drug levels have not been checked in a reasonable length of time, or when steps in a critical pathway must be taken. In general, they are triggered by a preceding event that starts a timer (for example, the order for a drug that needs monitoring of levels). If the timer expires before some canceling event occurs (an order for drug levels), the intervention is presented at the start of the ordering session or asynchronously.

Order sets and templates offer a menu of recommended orders based on a specific diagnosis, condition, or situation. The recommended orders have been compiled by a group of experts in the clinical domain. Order sets make it easy for the admitting doctor to execute these expert, optimized care plans. Because the use of sets and templates considerably reduces the time spent entering orders, this capability is an important component of a user-friendly POE system. In one report, 33 percent of all orders were entered through sets.[11] Algorithms represent an advanced special case of this class. Actions are generated based on a series of logical steps, as opposed to restricting the logic to just a single step. Data to support the decisions in the algorithm's flowchart can come from the clinical database or from the ordering physician directly in response to on-screen questionnaire forms. Standard structures for algorithms have been proposed[23] and practical applications of algorithms in POE are starting to appear.[24]

Rule-based event processing can be used to handle complex decision-support logic that does not fall into one of the above categories. In this class, rules written in a standard structure[25 26 15] are used to assess the current order in the light of other patient information—recent laboratory results, problem-list items, the patient's diet, admission status. Because of the general nature of this class, the trigger location and the action items are usually specified with the individual rule itself.

Rules Governance

Medical and administrative leaders are quick to recognize the power of clinical decision support. As initial interventions demonstrate success in changing physician behavior, they may seek to use this technology increasingly to solve clinical and resource-utilization problems. However, there are limits to the number of interventions that can be effectively implemented. If every order is accompanied by a series of warning screens, physicians are likely to react negatively to the extra time spent and the loss of independence. They may start to ignore all warning screens, finding ways to bypass them as quickly as possible; or they may become hostile to the continued use of the system altogether. The problem is exacerbated when interventions are imposed by one group on another without full communication about why the intervention is (or is not) appropriate.

Additionally, within a type of rule, the initial set of instances requiring intervention may be overstated. A common example is drug-drug checking. Drug manufacturers are motivated, if not required, to report any suspected interaction regardless of severity. These reports are faithfully included in commercial drug-interaction databases. However, a substantial number of these interactions may be of little clinical consequence. It may be necessary to intelligently pare down the list of interactions that generate interventions in order to focus physician attention on the truly important ones.[27]

For these reasons, it is important for an institution to have a governing body or bodies for reviewing new proposed interventions and for deciding which requests should get priority. The panel may include members of a variety of disciplines (medicine, nursing, pharmacy, laboratory) as well as participants from information systems. In my institution, new requests are accepted from department chairs or from hospital care-improvement committees; along with an initial feasibility review by information systems, an appropriate knowledge-domain committee reviews the request. For example, proposed medication interventions are reviewed by a subgroup of the pharmacy and therapeutics committee. The exchange of ideas within this multidisciplinary group has frequently led to a revised intervention that is acceptable to all and is thus more likely to gain compliance in the field.

Impact

It is clear from my experience and the experience of others that CDS aimed at POE may have a profound impact on a variety of care outcomes and cost. I will review how this impact has been assessed in a variety of studies and give an overview of the results of such studies.

Measurement. Decision support in POE is intended to prevent adverse events, to promote optimal care patterns, and to reduce excess utilization. Direct measurement of these variables is the most valuable way to assess the impact of a POE system. Measurement has been applied to the effect of a single intervention on a specific process, such as the use of target medications,[18] by looking at pharmacy distribution records. An intervention to promote appropriate antibiotic use[22] has relied on measurement of overall antibiotic costs and infection rates. Larger, carefully planned studies, including comprehensive chart review, have demonstrated the impact of POE on overall adverse drug events[12] and inpatient costs.[8] Chart review with a standardized data-entry form has also been used for a major study on the potential of information systems for detecting and preventing adverse events.[28]

Order entry creates its own database; about three thousand to eight thousand orders are generated for each inpatient bed per year. This large volume of data can be used to analyze compliance with the system's recommendations.

At one center, the rule editor can automatically be set to randomize a new intervention by patient or by doctor;[29] the impact is measured by comparing the ordering data of the control and the test groups.

Results. Published reports of specific care-improvement or cost-reduction interventions have generally shown a significant positive impact for POE.[30 8 12 18 21] Although there may be publication bias toward positive results, there are certainly many examples of dramatic behavioral change immediately following the institution of a new POE intervention. Some studies cite the prevention of hundreds of adverse events per year or annual cost savings in six figures with single interventions.

Success is more likely if the intervention is easy to understand, if action items are easy for the physician to select, and if the recommended ordering change is noncontroversial. In this ideal case, the computer is simply providing a just-in-time reminder of a fact that the physician had ignored or forgotten. Compliance is naturally lower when ordering physicians might disagree with the recommendation. A low compliance rate may indicate that the recommendation needs to be modified clinically or that more communication needs to take place between the clinical advocates of the intervention and the front-line physicians entering the orders.

Liability. Because POE systems recommend changes in therapeutic decisions, several legal questions arise. Is malpractice liability increased if the physician overrides a recommendation? Is the physician's liability decreased if he or she follows an incorrect recommendation? A related question is whether the system vendor incurs liability if its recommendations are incorrect or if it fails to generate an intervention where one would have been expected based on its prior performance.

All these issues ask the same question, which is whether the physician has a right (or a responsibility) to trust the computer. Many systems issue standard disclaimers stating that the final decision rests with the physician, and they back up that claim by requiring the physician to approve or reject all recommendations. Although this may be a valid legal position as well, the issue has not been extensively tested. At any rate, a convincing argument can be made that overall risk is reduced with a POE system because it catches errors and reduces adverse events in the first place.

Effect on Learning. A frequent question is whether exposure to POE with decision support during residency enhances or hinders a young doctor's education.[31] Anecdotal evidence suggests that residents who train with POE may not learn parameters (doses, frequencies) as well, but they learn to recognize hazardous situations better and are more familiar with standard or optimal paths of care. The reason presumably is that POE's just-in-time interventions educate the resident about a clinical situation precisely when the resident is focused on that situation (because it affects the resident's patient). This is an ideal time to learn information that will be retained.[32] Overall, educational effect is difficult to test because of the many other variables that affect residency training. Randomizing doctors to receive or not receive intervention messages could help answer the question, but at the expense of control-group patients who do not get the benefit of the interventions during the study period.

In any event, POE is not the first technology to be the subject of this concern. The question was raised when new diagnostic studies, particularly the computed-tomography scanner, were invented. Prior to that, some physicians even felt that diagnostic acumen would be destroyed by the introduction of arterial blood-gas testing, which is such a routine part of acute medical care today.[33] If POE systems become as universal as these technologies are, the question will become moot.

Conclusions

Many important decisions in acute medical care are expressed as inpatient orders. POE is a potent force for change because it can affect these orders at the source, communicating expert thought and current relevant data to the ordering provider. Published work from academic medical centers has demonstrated impressive benefits to quality of care and cost reduction through POE. However, a system's effectiveness and acceptance are quite sensitive to a number of factors. Intuitive design, attention to a priori leadership buy-in, capable implementation planning, and attentive support at start-up are important steps in bringing POE into an institution.

Once system acceptance has been attained, many interventions can be brought to bear on the ordering process. Introduction of new interventions is easiest when they are based on standard paradigms; development is then reduced to modifying a table or structure instead of requiring new programming from the institution or the vendor. An organized system of rules governance is valuable when a successful POE system starts to generate more and more requests for new interventions.

Future trends will likely include a greater emphasis on disease management and automatic selection of algorithms and protocols as well as more sophisticated rules and logic as additional types of clinical data become available in coded form.

References

1. Overhage, J. M., Tierney, W. M., Zhou, X. H., and McDonald, C. J. "A Randomized Trial of Corollary Orders to Prevent Errors of Omission." *Journal of American Medical Informatics Association*, 1997, *4* (5), 364–375.
2. Collen, M. F. "General Requirements for a Medical Information System (MIS)." *Computer Biomedical Research*, 1970, *3*, 393–406.
3. Dambro, M. R., Weiss, B. D., McClure, C. L., and Vuturo, A. F. "An Unsuccessful Experience with Computerized Medical Records in an Academic Medical Center." *Journal of Medical Education*, 1988, *63*, 617–623.

 4. Williams, L. S. "Microchips versus Stethoscopes: Calgary Hospital MDs Face Off Over Controversial Computer System." *Canadian Medical Association Journal*, 1992, *147*, 1535–1547.
 5. Massaro, T. A. "Introducing Physician Order Entry at a Major Academic Medical Center: Impact on Organizational Culture and Behavior." *Academy of Medicine*, 1993, *68*, 20–25.
 6. Sittig, D. F., and Stead, W. W. "Computer-Based Physician Order Entry: The State of the Art." *Journal of American Medical Informatics Association*, 1994, *1*(2), 108–123.
 7. McDonald, C. J. *Action-Oriented Decisions in Ambulatory Medicine.* Chicago: Year Book Medical Publishers, 1981.
 8. Tierney, W. M., Miller, M. E., Overhage, J. M., and McDonald, C. J. "Physician Inpatient Order Writing on Microcomputer Workstations: Effects on Resource Utilization." *Journal of the American Medical Association*, 1993, *269*, 379–383.
 9. Gardner, R. M., and others. "Computer-Critiqued Blood Ordering Using the HELP System." *Computer Biomedical Research*, 1990, *23*, 514–528.
10. Teich, J. M., Hurley, J. F., Beckley, R. F., and Aranow, M. "Design of an Easy-to-Use Physician Order Entry System with Support for Nursing and Ancillary Departments." *Proceedings of the Annual Symposium of Computer Applied Medical Care*, 1992, *16*, 99–103.
11. Teich, J. M., and others. "Toward Cost-Effective Quality Care: The Brigham Integrated Computing System." *Proceedings of the 2nd Nicholas E. Davies CPR Recognition Symposium.* Chicago: Computer-Based Patient Record Institute, 1996, 3–34.
12. Bates, D. W., and others. "Effect of Computerized Physician Order Entry and a Team Intervention on Prevention of Serious Medication Errors." *Journal of the American Medical Association*, 1998, *280* (15), 1311–1316.
13. Geissbuhler, A., Miller, R. A. "A New Approach to the Implementation of Direct Care-Provider Order Entry." *Journal of American Medical Informatics Association*, 1996, *3* (supplement), 689–693.
14. Ash, J. S., Horman, P. N., and Hersh, W. R. "Physician Order Entry in U. S. Hospitals." *Journal of American Medical Informatics Association*, 1998, *5* (supplement), 235–239.
15. Kuperman, G. J., and others. "Detecting Alerts, Notifying the Physician, and Offering Action Items: A Comprehensive Alerting System." *Journal of American Medical Informatics Association*, 1996, *3*(supplement), 704–708.
16. Teich, J. M., and others. "An Information System to Improve the Safety and Efficiency of Chemotherapy Ordering." *Journal of American Medical Informatics Association*, 1996, *3*(supplement), 498–502.
17. Teich, J. M., Kuperman, G. J., and Bates, D. W. "Transitioning Clinical Decision Support from the Hospital to the Community Network." *Healthcare Information Management*, 1997, *11* (4), 27–37.
18. Reynolds, M. S., and others. "Effect of an Education Computer Screen on Direct Physician Order Entry of Anti-Aerobic Drugs." *Proceedings of the 23rd Annual American Society of Hospitals and Pharmacies Mid-Year Clinical Meeting*, Dallas, TX, 1988.
19. Perry, M., and Myers, C. E. "Computer Cost Prompting as a Determinant of Hospital Drug Prescribing." *Proceedings of the 18th Annual American Society of Hospitals and Pharmacies Mid-Year Clinical Meeting*, Atlanta, GA, 1983.
20. Halpern, N. A., Thompson, R. E., and Greenstein, R. J. "A Computerized Intensive Care Unit Order-Writing Protocol." *Annual Review of Pharmacology*, 1992, *26*, 251–254.
21. Harpole, L. H., and others. "Automated Evidence-Based Critiquing of Orders for Abdominal Radiographs: Impact on Utilization and Appropriateness." *Journal of American Medical Informatics Association*, 1997, *4* (6), 511–521.
22. Pestotnik, S. L., Classen, D. C., Evans, R. S., and Burke, J. P. "Implementing Antibiotic Practice Guidelines through Computer-Assisted Decision Support: Clinical and Financial Outcomes." *Annals of Internal Medicine*, 1996, *124* (10), 884–890.
23. Ohno-Machado, L., and others. "The Guideline Interchange Format: A Model for Representing Guidelines." *Journal of American Medical Informatics Association*, 1998, *5* (4), 357–372.

24. Zielstorff, R. D., "Online Practical Guidelines: Issues, Obstacles, and Future Prospects." *Journal of American Medical Informatics Association*, 1998, *5* (3), 227–236.

25. Pryor, T. A., and Hripcsak, G. "The Arden Syntax for Medical Logic Modules." *International Journal of Clinical Monitoring and Computing*, 1993, *10* (4), 215–224.

26. Overhage, J. M., and others. "A Tool for Provider Interaction During Patient Care: G-CARE." *Journal of American Medical Informatics Association*, 1995, 2(supplement), 178–182.

27. Paterno, M. D., Teich, J. M., Seger, D. L., and Bates, D. W. "A Practical Method for Presenting Drug Interactions to Clinicians." *Journal of American Medical Informatics Association*, 1996, *3*(supplement), 872.

28. Bates, D. W., and others. "Potential Identifiability and Preventability of Adverse Events Using Information Systems." *Journal of American Medical Informatics Association*, 1994, *1* (5), 404–411.

29. Kuperman, G. J., and others. "Representing Hospital Events as Complex Conditionals." *Journal of American Medical Informatics Association*, 1995, 2(supplement), 137–141.

30. Hunt, D. L., Haynes, R. B., Hanna, S. E., and Smith, K. "Effects of Computer-Based Decision Support Systems on Physician Performance and Patient Outcomes: A Systematic Review." *Journal of the American Medical Association*, 1998, *280* (15), 1339–1346.

31. Stair, T. O., and Howell, J. M. "Effect on Medical Education of Computerized Physician Order Entry." *Academic Medicine*, 1995, *70* (6), 543.

32. Chueh, H., and Barnett, G. O. "Just-in-Time Clinical Information." *Acad Med*, 1997, *72* (6), 512–517.

33. Braunwald, E. M., personal communication.

About the Author

Jonathan M. Teich, M.D., Ph.D., is corporate director for clinical-systems research and development at Partners HealthCare System, the network formed by Massachusetts General Hospital and Brigham and Women's Hospital in Boston. He is also an attending physician in emergency medicine at Brigham and Women's.

Design and Architecture
of Asynchronous Push Technology
for Clinical Decision Support

Homer R. Warner, Jr., M.S.; Di Guo, Ph.D.;
Christopher Mason; William Harty; Lili Li, M.S.

Acknowledgments: Development of the Clinical Event Manager was funded jointly by a Department of Commerce NIST ATP Grant (95-10) and Sunquest Information Systems, Inc., of Tucson, Arizona.

Since 1970, several computer-based clinical decision support systems have been successfully implemented in hospital settings.[1][2][3][4] These systems analyze patient information, identify significant trends, and attempt to ensure that important information is presented to the health provider at the point of care. However, the benefit and use of these sophisticated real-time decision-support systems have been limited largely to the care providers and healthcare settings where computers play an integral part in healthcare delivery.

The widespread use of real-time clinical alerting has been limited by several factors:

The cost of replacing legacy systems. Sophisticated decision-support systems have been "closed systems" lacking the modularity that would make them portable without requiring an information-system overhaul for the buyer.

Inflexible system architecture. Rigidity in programming languages, databases, knowledge bases, and alert delivery have historically limited users' control over alert selection, timing, and delivery methods.

Limited asynchronous options for alert and reminder notification for non-computer and mobile users.

To address these concerns, we developed the modular, computer-based Clinical Event Manager, called CEM. CEM is a real-time, asynchronous push technology that "listens in" on the hospital's Health Level Seven (HL7) event traffic. It filters the clinical data through an inference engine that looks for selected critical events in laboratory, pharmacy, demographic, and radiologic information and then broadcasts vital patient data (for example, alerts and reminders) to caregivers by way of alphanumeric pagers or e-mail (or both).

The CEM project began in September 1995 and is now operational at six sites. The University of Utah Medical Center (UUMC), a 400-bed teaching and level-one trauma center in Salt Lake City, was the first site to "go live" with CEM, in May 1997. Five others followed, completing implementations in 1998. The implementation and evaluations of CEM at these sites are described elsewhere.[5] In this article, we describe the design and architecture of CEM.

CEM consists of four major modules, which play keys roles in the successful operation of the system: the run-time components, the subscription module, the module for provider-patient coverage, and the dictionary and rule editor. The server-based run-time components are the workhorse of the system and provide nonstop collecting, filtering, storing, and broadcasting of vital clinical messages to subscribers in real time.

Run-Time Components

CEM's run-time components utilize Microsoft's Component Object Model (COM). COM is a component software architecture that allows applications and systems to be built from components supplied by different software vendors. CEM has seven COM/ActiveX servers (square boxes) as shown in Figure 1. The information flows through CEM via COM interfaces among different components, using data-container components and data-access components.

The CEM run-time application is divided into different logical components so that changes can be made to a specific component without having to change the entire system. CEM's COM components are written in a mixture of C++, Visual Basic, and Java programming languages. CEM's database schema is tailored for the rapid data-retrieval needs of the inference engine.

CEM processes events in one of two modes: a data-driven mode, where rules are triggered by a new piece of data, such as a new laboratory result; or a time-driven mode, where a task is scheduled to be run at a certain time as a result of a clinical event (for example, "whenever the drug gentamicin is prescribed, check for the drug level after forty-eight hours").

In the data-driven mode, CEM acquires clinical events through an HL7 interface engine. HL7 messages are parsed, coded, and then stored in CEM's SQL Server relational database. Clinical data are coded based on CEM's dictionary tables in the database. Data-integrity rules are implemented through stored procedures to flag any invalid data such as data correction and multiple transmission of the same laboratory result.

After data are stored in CEM's database, they are passed along to the inference engine (developed using COM components from Neuron Data Elements Expert) to determine whether they meet the criteria for any rules in CEM's knowledge base. If a data item satisfies the logic of a rule, an output is

Figure 1. Process Flow for the Clinical Event Manager

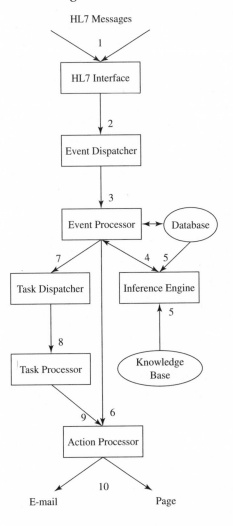

1. HL7 Interface intercepts HL7 messages from different systems (e.g., lab, pharmacy, patient registration) on a network, parses them, and stores patient data into SQL Server.
2. Event Dispatcher gets notified whenever new information is available and maintains an event queue.
3. Events are pushed one by one from Event Dispatcher to Event Processor.
4. Event Processor retrieves patient information associated with an event and sends it to the Inference Engine for analysis.
5. The Inference Engine invokes relevant rules. It retrieves additional patient data from the database and knowledge base if needed (e.g., additional lab results for trending) and returns reminders or alerts to Event Processor.
6. Event Processor receives output from the Inference Engine and pushes it to Action Processor.
7. Tasks can be scheduled from the Inference Engine as the result of a clinical event. Event Processor pushes tasks into Task Dispatcher.
8. Task Dispatcher pushes a task that is due to run to Task Processor.
9. Task Processor generates reminders or alerts and pushes them to Action Processor.
10. Action Processor processes inferences and delivers them to subscribers through e-mail or pagers.

generated from the inference engine. COM interfaces are provided for accessing different states of business objects during an inference session, which makes alert objects generated by Neuron Data's inference engine easily accessible by CEM's event processor. The inference output is then relayed on to the action processor, which handles message deployment.

A strength of this system is its ability to deliver critical information how, where, and when the caregiver desires. CEM can deliver information via pager, e-mail, fax, and printer. Pagers and e-mail have been the most widely used asynchronous method of information deployment. The CEM system uses Microsoft's

Messaging API to communicate with any back-end messaging services. This interface supports popular e-mail systems like cc:Mail and GroupWise.

For paging services, CEM uses standard interfaces such as e-mail gateways and Telocator Alphanumeric Protocol (TAP). Custom protocols can also be implemented. CEM supports three kinds of alphanumeric pagers:

One-way pagers receive messages but fail if the user is in a "dead zone" such as a building basement.

Guaranteed-delivery pagers, in which the paging device acknowledges to the transmitter receipt of a message. The transmitter will retransmit any failed messages until it is successful.

Two-way pagers offer guaranteed delivery plus the ability to acknowledge messages.

To ensure patient-data confidentiality, CEM supports protocols such as HTTPS, MIME/S, and private key encryption provided by Microsoft's MAPI services. Security can be further enhanced by using private point-to-point network connections to paging and e-mail services through leased lines. However, the security of patient data is also dependent on the security provided by a hospital's network infrastructure and the security provided by the paging and e-mail providers.

Subscription Module

Healthcare providers subscribe to the system by completing either a paper-based or computer-based subscription form that lists rules and subscription properties. Exhibit 1 is a portion of the subscription form. The subscription module is used to store the user's preferences in CEM's database. The broadcasting module (action processor) relies on this information to determine message routing. Subscribers can specify times when the alert should be

Exhibit 1. Subscription Form for Specifying Preferences

Rule Name	Description	New Threshold	Send Times:	Only Send When:	Method
ABG: Critical value	ABG with (Ph < 7.25) or (Po2 < 50) or (Pco2 > 50)	New threshold:	__ Send every time it triggers __ Only send 1st time __ Send after __ days	Only send days: __ Only send	Pager E-mail Printer
ABGs	Arterial Blood Gas results.	New threshold:	__ Send every time it triggers __Only send 1st time __ Send after __ days	Only send days: __ Only send	Pager E-mail Printer

delivered ("send alerts to my pager only between 9:00 A.M. and 5:00 P.M., but send to my e-mail at all times"). Subscribers can choose to receive an alert every time it triggers for a specific patient ("notify every time potassium is elevated") or just when the alert is triggered the first time ("notify only the first time the patient's creatinine is elevated"). Subscribers can choose to receive the first alert and then receive it again only after three days if the condition is still met ("notify of a drug interaction between Amiodarone and Coumadin once, but alert again after three days if the problem persists"). The subscription module can also be used to request a new threshold for an existing rule.

Module for Provider-Patient Coverage

Perhaps the biggest challenge in implementing CEM was in figuring out provider-patient coverage, or to whom to send the alert. CEM accommodates sending alerts under these circumstances:

- For any patient where the subscriber is an attending or ordering physician
- For patients on a particular service or nursing unit
- For every patient in the hospital for certain indicators
- For selected patients chosen via the hospital information system for grouping laboratories
- For patients selected using CEM's coverage module

CEM's coverage module enables clinicians to identify and group the patients they are covering. Subscribers spend an average of ten minutes to set up their initial patient list and then approximately three minutes a day to maintain the list. The coverage module has team-support features that reduce maintenance. For example, an attending physician may have many patients being seen by residents, interns, and students. This hierarchy eliminates redundant coverage-list entry.

Coverage-list maintenance can be centralized where caregivers phone in, e-mail, fax, or print their patient lists to a central location for entry into CEM. If subscribers are already maintaining their patient lists on a hospital information system, an interface can be developed to populate CEM's coverage list automatically. Coverage interfaces to CEM were developed for UUMC and MCMH.

Rule and Dictionary Editing

Tools have been created to develop and maintain CEM's knowledge base of four hundred rules and the supporting dictionary of six thousand terms. These tools enable the creation and modification of the three major elements in the knowledge base: classes and objects, database access, and rules. Objects are the building blocks for rules. For example, the platelet-count object is used in a "low platelet rule" and in an adverse drug event rule like "NSAIDS [nonsteroidal anti-inflammatory drugs] and low platelet count." Objects are related to classes through a hierarchical network. For example, a class called "Medication" defines a medication order. This class has properties such as "Status" (active or inactive) whose value is determined from the medication table in the database. Once a property is defined, it can be inherited by any specific medication object attached to the "Medication" class. Database access facilitates the development of rules, which can consist of interdisciplinary data sources (for example, drug and laboratory) as well as data from multiple observation points over time for trending. CEM rules use a simple symbolic syntax ("if Med.Status = 'Active' then alert").

System Management

Most of CEM's administration processes are automated. CEM is self-monitoring. On a regular schedule, a central monitoring module, named Console, communicates with the Windows NT operating system to determine whether each of CEM's core components is in memory. Console also regularly sends a custom HL7 message through CEM and waits for a test alert to come out the other end. This "loop-back test" is an excellent system-monitoring device because it will succeed only if each CEM component is operating correctly. Console sends administrator alerts out via e-mail or pager or both. Periodic pages can also be sent to the systems administrator (SA) indicating that everything is all right. If a page is not received within a predefined time interval the SA knows that CEM needs to be checked.

CEM uses a database backup scheme that maximizes run time efficiency and minimizes recovery time. The database is completely backed up every other day, and the database transaction logs are backed up four times a day. In the event of a system failure, the database is restored from the most recent backup, all transaction logs since that backup are applied, and, if needed, the HL7 messages processed since the last recorded transaction are fed through CEM.

CEM uses an "aging" process to clear up data periodically for system performance and ease of maintenance. The general rule is that a patient's clinical data are deleted if the patient is discharged from the hospital or if the data are more than 120 days old. Patient and provider demographic data are not deleted because of their slow growth in volume. Some clinical data—such as a positive Vancomycin Resistant Enterococcus (VRE) culture—are not aged because of inference needs—the culture result is required for checking readmission of a patient with VRE history.

System Configuration and Performance

CEM runs on Microsoft BackOffice 2.5, which includes Windows NT Server 4.0, SQL Server 6.5, and Internet Information Server 5.0. CEM's base system has dual 300MHz Pentium II processors, 256MB RAM, 9GB of Fast-Wide SCSI RAID5 disk space with a hot spare (four drives total), 24GB DDS tape backup, and a redundant power supply. This system can be scaled up to eight processors, 4GB RAM for large or multifacility sites.

Using this hardware configuration at UUMC and MCMH, CEM processes 2.5 million and 4.7 million HL7 messages and events per year, respectively. CEM's performance is measured in terms of its ability to process inbound HL7 messages and send outbound alerts. Central-processing-unit and disk performance affect inbound performance, while network latency (e-mail and paging services) affects outbound performance. CEM subscribers typically receive their alerts via pager or e-mail within three minutes of CEM's receiving and processing the HL7 message or event.

Discussion

The installations of CEM at both UUMC and MCMH left the legacy information systems intact and required interfaces only between the hospital HL7 gateway and CEM. This was an important step in accomplishing our goal of building an adaptable alerting and reminding system that could fit into any HL7-compliant legacy-system environment. Because e-mail and paging methods for information deployment are available through CEM, healthcare providers now have an alternative to synchronous messaging. This text paging method provides a needed option for providers who do not use computers or who use them infrequently and for anyone who prefers a combination of push-pull technology.

We anticipate that paging methods will become even more acceptable with the advent of paging devices with larger display screens, like 3Com PalmPilot. As others are finding who are working with asynchronous decision-support technology,[6] much remains to be learned about the use of bidirectional paging, which holds promise of making CEM-like systems become mission-critical applications. In addition, more work needs to be done to devise simpler methods for identifying physician-patient coverage.

References

1. Haug, P. J., and others. "Decision Support in Medicine: Examples from the HELP System." *Computers and Biomedical Research,* 1994, 27, 396–418.
2. McDonald, C. J., Tierney, W. M., Martin, D. K., and Overhage, J. M. "The Regenstrief Medical Record System: 20 Years of Experience in Hospitals, Clinics and Neighborhood Health Centers." *MD Computing,* 1992, 9 (4), 206–217.
3. Jenders, R. A., and others. "Medical Decision Support: Experience with Implementing the Arden Syntax at the Columbia-Presbyterian Medical Center." *Proceedings of the Annual Symposium on Computer Applications in Medical Care,* 1995, 19, 169–173.
4. Kuperman, G. J., and others. "Detecting Alerts, Notifying the Physician, and Offering Action Items: A Comprehensive Alerting System." *Proceedings of the American Medical Informatics Association Annual Fall Symposium,* 1996, 704–708.

5. Warner, H. R., Jr., and others. "Clinical Event Management Using Push Technology—Implementation and Evaluation at Two Health Care Centers." *Proceedings of the American Medical Informatics Association Annual Fall Symposium,* 1998, 106–110.
6. Wagner, M. M., and others. "Clinical Event Monitoring at the University of Pittsburgh." *Proceedings of the American Medical Informatics Association Annual Fall Symposium,* 1997, 188–192.

About the Authors

Homer R. Warner, Jr., M.S. is a doctoral candidate at the Department of Medical Informatics of the University of Utah.

Di Guo, Ph.D., is the principal software developer for Sunquest Information Systems, Salt Lake City, Utah.

Christopher Mason is director of software development at Sunquest Information Systems, Salt Lake City, Utah.

William Harty is senior software developer at Sunquest Information Systems, Salt Lake City, Utah.

Lili Li, M.S., is a software developer at Sunquest Information Systems, Salt Lake City, Utah.

To order: Contact HIMSS, (312) 664-HIMSS (4467); web site: http://www. himss.org; or fax on demand: 1-800-HIMSS-11 (1-800-446-7711). Also contact HIMSS for more information about additional HIMSS resources for the healthcare information and management systems professional.

Books

Guide to Effective Healthcare Information and Management Systems and the Role of the CIO is a complete revision of the 1994 publication. Outlining the changing roles and responsibilities of CIOs as well as providing solutions by industry leaders, this revision addresses how the role of the CIO has changed. 232 pages.

Price: HIMSS members $15; non-members $22
(Volume discounts available on 25 or more)

Guide to Effective Health Care Telecommunications discusses the role and organization of telecommunications management including a historical perspective, strategic planning, enabling technologies, and needs analysis. 140 pages.

Price: HIMSS members $10; non-members $15
(Volume discounts available on 25 or more)

Guide to Effective Health Care Management Engineering explains the crucial role of the management engineer in health care today, and presents the tools and techniques that make the management engineer a critical team member. 34 pages.

Price: HIMSS members $10; non-members $15
(Volume discounts available on 25 or more)

Guide to Nursing Informatics provides a glossary of terms and key concepts that can be used as preparation for the American Nurses' Credentialing Center (ANCC) certification exam or as a reference for practicing nurses. 25 pages.

Price: HIMSS members $10; non-members $15
(Volume discounts available on 25 or more)

Conference Proceedings

Proceedings of the 1999 Annual HIMSS Conference and Exhibition (Atlanta, GA), 4-volume boxed set, approximately 1,500 pages, 144 educational sessions, and 36 poster presentations.

Price: HIMSS members $65; non-members $95
CD-ROM/Proceedings of the 1999 Annual HIMSS Conference and Exhibition (Atlanta, GA), fully searchable/retrievable text and graphics of the technical presentations, attendee roster, and poster presentation.

Price: HIMSS members $90; non-members $135

Proceedings of the 1998 Annual HIMSS Conference and Exhibition (Orlando, FL), 4-volume boxed set, approximately 1,500 pages, 157 educational sessions, and 17 poster presentations.

Price: HIMSS members $45; non-members $65

CD-ROM/Proceedings of the 1998 Annual HIMSS Conference and Exhibition (Orlando, FL), fully searchable/retrievable text and graphics of the technical presentations, attendee roster, and poster presentations.

Price: HIMSS members $65; non-members $95

Audio/Visual

Selected sessions for HIMSS educational events are available from ACTS INC., (314) 394-0611, fax (314) 394-9381.

Writer's Guidelines

Journal of Healthcare Information Management® (*JHIM*) is a quarterly peer-reviewed journal devoted to professional development issues in healthcare information and management systems. It is published by the Healthcare Information and Management Systems Society, Chicago, a not-for-profit membership organization dedicated to the promotion of better understanding of healthcare information and management systems and to the professional growth of its members.

Readership and Circulation

JHIM® circulation is approximately 12,000. The primary audience includes professionals in hospital administration, information systems, management engineering, telecommunications, clinical professions, consultants, university program faculty, and managers in other sectors of the healthcare field. *JHIM*® is indexed by the American Hospital Association's Hospital Literature Index and the National Library of Medicine's on-line bibliographic database, *Health*.

Manuscript Submission

JHIM® seeks articles in the following formats:

- *Market Analysis:* Articles defining the state of the field, or its various components, and identifying their information and management system needs.
- *Technology Overview:* Articles surveying and defining the key enabling technologies and business methodologies for the field or its components (mobile computing, relational databases, handwriting/voice recognition, and so on); formulas for budgeting and needs assessment.
- *Case Studies:* Articles explaining who, what, when, how, and why of a particular problem or challenge, and how it was solved or solution proposal.
- *Book/Literature/Resource Review:* In-depth articles reviewing a book or resource (including on-line products and services). Articles surveying a variety of resources to further readers' understanding of the field.

  Authors should submit a one-page proposal including the following information:
- One- to two-paragraph abstract
- Complete name, title, address, telephone number, fax number, and e-mail address of all potential authors

Send to Julie Foreman, Manager, Editorial Services, HIMSS, 230 E. Ohio St., Suite 500, Chicago, IL 60611-3269. You will be contacted upon acceptance of the article.

Manuscript Preparation

Length
- 3,000 to 5,000 words, single-spaced, excluding figures, tables, and appendixes
- Author biographies are limited to 30 words and should appear at the end of text

Layout
- Use standard sized 8½" × 11" white paper with one-inch margins on all sides.
- Use single column format, single-spaced, ragged right.

Font
- Use 10-point type for body copy. Serif fonts such as Palatino or Times Roman are preferred.
- Text included in charts, graphs, and figures should be as large as possible to maximize readability.

Headings
- DO NOT include an abstract at the beginning of the paper.
- DO NOT leave blank pages or columns within the document.
- DO NOT start each new section on a new page.
- Major headings should be in CAPITAL LETTERS, 12 point, flush left within the column. Please DO NOT bold.
- Subheadings should be in upper and lowercase, 10 point, flush left within the column on a separate line following paragraph. Please DO NOT bold.
- Sub-subheadings should be in upper and lowercase, 10 point, flush left within the column at the beginning of the paragraph. They may be either bold or italicized to set off title from body text.

Figures/Graphs/Charts
- Limit the number of figures, graphs, and charts to three.
- Assign a title and figure number to each.
- In text, refer to all figures, graphs, and charts by title and figure number.
- Label x and y axis of every graph.
- Distinguish bars or pie chart sections by pattern, not color.
- DO NOT INCLUDE graphics in the computer file version of the paper. Save all graphics in a separate text file. Use the figure title and number for file name.
- DO INCLUDE two hard copies of each graphic (if graphics are not retrievable they will be scanned).

File Format

Required Media: Mac 3.5″ 1.4MB or 800K or PC/Win 3.5″ 1.4 MB

Provide text as straight text, following the minimal formatting guidelines previously stated. Save figures and graphics in a separate text file. Page breaks, bolding, underlining, italicizing, and so on, are strongly discouraged. Save each figure and graph as a separate document. The original hard copy layout of the document will be used as a reference.

Acceptable file formats (text only):
Word processors:

Mac	PC
Word	Text
Excel	RTF
Powerpoint	Word (DOS and Windows)
Photoshop	WordPerfect (DOS and Windows)
Quark	
Pagemaker	
Claris Works	

Note: If using Windows, please save in Word 6.0 or lower.
Acceptable file formats (graphics):

Mac (PICT) to PC	PC to Mac (PICT)
TIFF	PC Paintbrush.PCX
Windows Bitmap.BMP	TIFF
Windows Metafile.WMF	Windows.BMP

Electronic Submission

Manuscripts that do not contain figures or graphs may be submitted via e-mail. Send to jforeman@himss.org.

Style and Presentation

- Use standard spelling, style, reference, and grammar guides such as *Webster's New Collegiate Dictionary, American Medical Association Manual of Style,* and *The Elements of Style.*
- Use active sentences and be specific. Back up generalities with examples. Avoid jargon.
- All articles will be copyedited and, where necessary, rewritten. The process by which authors may review and approve changes is defined in the letter of agreement.

References

- Submit only complete references.
- In the text body, numbers should appear in square brackets [1]. In the reference list, numbers should be in bullet format.
- Use AMA style for references. Please refer to the following:

Books:
1. Foreman, J. F., and Fulkerson, W. F. (1997). *HIMSS Writer's Guidelines.* Chicago: Healthcare Information and Management Systems Society.

Periodicals:
2. Gabriel, D. (1996). "New Team, New Look." *HIMSS News,* 6 (12), 10–12.

- Reference list should begin on a separate page following the document.
- References should be numbered and listed in the text body in order of appearance.

Submission Checklist

- Manuscript on 3.5″ Macintosh or PC disk following formatting guidelines
- One hard copy, formatted with art and figures
- Two (2) separate copies of each piece of art
- Signed letter of agreement

HEALTHCARE INFORMATION AND MANAGEMENT SYSTEMS SOCIETY

The Healthcare Information and Management Systems Society (HIMSS) provides leadership in healthcare for the management of systems, information, and change. Its more than 12,000 professional members include individuals in the fields of clinical systems, information systems, management engineering, and telecommunications working in healthcare organizations throughout the world and dedicated to promoting a better understanding of healthcare information and management systems.

HIMSS performs and publishes research in key areas including the HIMSS Annual Leadership Survey on trends in healthcare computing and the Annual HIMSS Compensation Study. In addition, HIMSS sponsors the most comprehensive annual conference and exhibition in this field, as well as numerous regional educational events.

For more information about membership, publications, and educational events, contact HIMSS at 312/664-HIMSS (4467), Web Site: http://www.himss.org, E-mail: himss@himss.org, or Fax-on-Demand Document Service: 800/HIMSS-11 (800/446-7711).

1999–2000 HIMSS Officers

President
Jeffrey Cooper, FHIMSS, Vice President, Ancillary Services and CIO, Henry Medical Center, Stockbridge, GA

President-Elect
Gary Kurtz, FHIMSS, System Officer—IT, PennState Geisinger Health System, Danville, PA

Vice President
Pamela Matthews, FHIMSS, Senior Management Consultant—IS Planning, Superior Consultant Company, Atlanta, GA

Vice President–Elect
Lavone C. Neal, FHIMSS, Vice President, Financial Analysis/Decision Support Services, Baylor Health Care System, Dallas, TX

1999–2000 HIMSS Directors

Nancy Aldrich, FHIMSS, President, Telecommunications Management Corporation, Waltham, MA

Wayne Anderson, FHIMSS, Director of Management Engineering, University of Alabama Hospital, Birmingham, AL

Sandra Bailey, FHIMSS, Administrator, Methodist Healthcare-Brownsville Hospital, Brownsville, TN

Pamela McNutt, Vice President, Systems and CIO, Methodist Hospital of Dallas, Dallas, TX

Walter R. Menning, Vice Chairman, Information Services, Mayo Foundation, Rochester, MN

Rosemary Nelson, Program Manager and CIO, Pacific Regional Program Office, Tripler Army Medical Center, HI

Linda Reeder, RN, CHE, Director of Marketing, Advanced Research Systems, Seattle, WA

Paul Vegoda, FHIMSS, Vice President and CIO, North Shore Health System, Great Neck, NY

HEALTHCARE INFORMATION AND MANAGEMENT SYSTEMS SOCIETY
PROFESSIONAL EDUCATIONAL EVENTS

Nursing Informatics Workshop
August 13–14, 1999—Cleveland, OH
October 15–16, 1999—Los Angeles, CA

Telehealth: Steps to Successful Implementation
September 23–25, 1999
Atlanta, GA

Improving Performance: Tools for Success Workshop
November 4–6, 1999
Dallas, TX

Long Term Care Information Systems Conference
September 13–15, 1999
Tampa, FL

Introduction to Healthcare Information Systems Workshop
September 30–October 2, 1999
Las Vegas, NV

All inquiries should be forwarded to:

Healthcare Information and Management Systems Society

mail: 230 East Ohio Street, Suite 500
        Chicago, IL 60611-3269

phone: (312) 664-HIMS (4467)

fax: (312) 664-6143

e-mail: himss@himss.org

web site: http://www.himss.org

fax-on-demand document service: 800/HIMSS-11 (800/446-7711)

Ordering Information

Journal of Healthcare Information Management®, published quarterly, is devoted to issues of significance in the professional development of individuals working in the areas of clinical systems, information systems, management engineering, and telecommunications.

Subscriptions cost $63.00 for individuals and $95.00 for institutions, agencies, and libraries. Standing orders are accepted. New York residents, add local sales tax. (For subscriptions outside the United States, orders must be prepaid in U.S. dollars by check drawn on a U.S. bank or charged to VISA, MasterCard, or American Express.)

Single copies cost $24.00 plus shipping (see below) when payment accompanies order. California, New Jersey, New York, and Washington, D.C., residents please include appropriate sales tax. Canadian residents, add GST and any local taxes. Billed orders will be charged shipping and handling. No billed shipments to post office boxes. (Orders from outside the United States must be prepaid in U.S. dollars by check drawn on a U.S. bank or charged to VISA, MasterCard, or American Express.)
Shipping (Single Copies Only): $30.00 and under, add $5.50; to $50, add $6.50; to $75.00, add $7.50; to $100, add $9.00; to $150.00, add $10.00.

Reprints of individual articles: For quantities of 25 and under, contact the Healthcare Information and Management Systems Society, 230 East Ohio Street, Suite 500, Chicago, IL 60611-3269. Phone: (312) 664-4467. For quantities over 25, contact Vincent Fritzsche, Jossey-Bass Publishers, 350 Sansome Street, San Francisco, CA 94104-1342. Phone: (415) 433-1740, extension 3198.

Microfilm copies of issues and articles are available in 16mm and 35mm, as well as microfiche in 105mm, through University Microfilms Inc., 300 North Zeeb Road, Ann Arbor, MI 48106-1346.

Discounts for quantity orders are available. Please write to the address below for information.

All orders must include either the name of an individual or an official purchase order number. Please submit your orders as follows:
Subscriptions: specify issue (for example, HCIM 10:1) you would like subscription to begin with.
Single copies: specify volume and issue number.

Mail orders to:
Jossey-Bass Publishers
350 Sansome Street
San Francisco, California 94104-1342

Phone subscription or single-copy orders toll-free at (800) 956-7739 or at (415) 433-1767

Fax orders toll-free to: (800) 605-2665

Librarians are encouraged to contact the Periodicals Marketing Department at Jossey-Bass Publishers for a free sample issue.

Visit the Jossey-Bass home page on the World Wide Web at www.josseybass.com for an order form or information about other titles of interest.